Fibromyalgia & Chronic Fatigue Syndrome

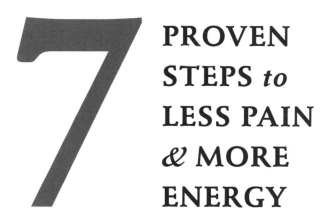

7 PROVEN STEPS *to* LESS PAIN *&* MORE ENERGY

FRED FRIEDBERG, PH.D.

New Harbinger Publications, Inc.

Distributed in Canada by Raincoast Books.

Copyright © 2006 by Fred Friedberg
New Harbinger Publications, Inc.
5674 Shattuck Avenue
Oakland, CA 94609
www.newharbinger.com

Cover design by Amy Shoup; Acquired by Jess O'Brien; Edited by Amy Johnson; Text design by Tracy Marie Carlson

---

Library of Congress Cataloging-in-Publication Data

Friedberg, Fred.
   Fibromyalgia and chronic fatigue syndrome : seven proven steps to less pain and more energy / Fred Friedberg.
       p. cm.
   ISBN-13: 978-1-57224-459-7
   ISBN-10: 1-57224-459-3
   1. Chronic fatigue syndrome—Popular works. 2. Fibromyalgia—Popular works. I. Title.
   RB150.F37F752 2006
   616'.0478—dc22

                                                    2006007021

08   07   06

10   9   8   7   6   5   4   3   2   1

First printing

To Pat and Mae

Contents

PART III
Physicians, Treatments, and "Cures"

Foreword

As Dr. Friedberg wisely notes in this excellent book, all illnesses, including heart attacks, cancers, and even schizophrenia have both a physical and psychological component—and are best healed when both of these are treated simultaneously. Chronic fatigue syndrome and fibromyalgia (CFS/FMS) are no exceptions. In the West, an inappropriate distinction has been made attempting to separate illnesses into being either physical or mental. In large part, this has occurred because insurance companies pay far less for what are considered psychological or mental illnesses and have therefore fought hard to inappropriately categorize CFS/FMS as a psychological disorder. While this categorization is used by the insurance companies as an excuse to not pay the billions of dollars that they owe patients, it comes at the expense of already devastated patients and is not just unethical and illegal but grossly inappropriate.

Our published "Gold Standard" double-blind placebo-controlled study has proven that CFS/FMS are real physical diseases. By treating patients using our SHIN protocol (addressing sleep, hormonal deficiencies, infections, and nutritional deficiencies), our study showed that 91 percent of CFS/FMS patients improve with an average increase in quality of life of 90 percent. The study also showed that psychoactive medications did not significantly improve patient outcomes. Besides showing that these are treatable syndromes, the study demonstrates that those who believe that they are all in your mind have gone from being nitwits to being unscientific nitwits! For those of you who would like to explore this further, the full text of the study can be seen at www.vitality101.com.

I know what you've been through. 1975 was a really rough year. I was caught in the middle of a family meltdown while in my third year of medical school. I was twenty-two, and my father had died years earlier, so I was paying my own way. Finally the stress caught up with me. I had what I called the "drop-dead flu." Three months later, I was still exhausted, unable to sleep, achy all over, and had no brain. Devastated, I had to drop out of medical school. As I was paying my own way and relying on scholarships, student loans, and work (which I was now too sick to do), I found myself homeless and sleeping in parks. This was to be my introduction to chronic fatigue syndrome and fibromyalgia.

CFS/FMS Triggers

I do not view these syndromes as the enemy. Rather, I see them as attempts on the body's part to protect itself from further harm and damage in the face of any of a number of overwhelming stresses. A simple way to look at fibromyalgia and CFS would be to view them like a circuit breaker in a house. When certain systems are overstressed, the circuit breaker will go off to prevent damage to the home's wiring. In milder cases, your body's circuit breaker can come back on and systems can return to healthy function by simply supplying the body with rest and proper nutrition. In CFS/FMS, however, it is as if the main circuit breaker (in this situation, the hypothalamus, a master gland in the brain) has turned off. When this occurs, rest is no longer enough to restore proper function.

Despite the many diverse triggers that can cause these syndromes, most patients' symptoms seem to come from a common endpoint— excessive energy demands resulting in dysfunction or suppression of the hypothalamic circuit breaker. This area controls sleep, hormonal function, temperature regulation, and the autonomic nervous system (blood pressure, blood flow, sweating, and movement of food through the bowel). The hypothalamic dysfunction by itself can therefore cause most of the symptoms we see in these patients.

Physical and Situational Stresses

As is the case with other illnesses (like heart attacks), the trigger can be physical and/or psychological stresses. In fact, anything that results in your overdrawing your "energy account" can trigger the process. Once you've blown the fuse, you're most likely to get well when you treat both the physical and psychological "energy drainers." While a number of books (including my book *From Fatigued to Fantastic*, 2001) expertly address how to treat the physical component of these syndromes, few thoroughly address the psycho-spiritual steps you can take to reclaim your health—an area you have full power over. In fact, in my experience, almost all illnesses have a psychodynamic that characterizes them.

The Psychodynamic of CFS/FMS

Having treated over 3000 patients with these syndromes, I have found that most people with CFS/FMS are mega-type-A overachievers. As a group, our sensitivity and intuitive abilities are high. We had low self-esteem as children and tended to seek approval, often from someone who simply was not going to give it. This, combined with our sensitivity to the feelings of others, caused us to avoid conflict and to try to meet other people's needs—at the expense of our own. Many of us closed off our feelings (and our empathic nature) for a while because we were too young to handle their intensity. Because of our approval seeking and low self-esteem, we often drove ourselves to being the best at what we did or to try to be all things to all people. Not being able to say no (because we wanted to avoid conflict or loss of approval) led us to feel as though we could not defend our emotional boundaries, which therefore left us feeling drained. We responded to fatigue by redoubling our efforts instead of resting, as our bodies (and the healthy signal called fatigue) tried to tell us to do. This contributed to our depleting our energy reserves—sometimes while feeling great on an adrenaline high. In addition, being people pleasers, have you ever noted how you seem to attract people who are "energy vampires" and leave you feeling even more drained?

By working on both my physical and psychological issues, I have achieved a full recovery. The illness actually became a blessing that taught me to get touch with my own feelings and desires. I live a very busy life now, but moving at optimal speed is a lot healthier if you are going in the right direction! Before you can do this, however, you have to know what you really want instead of seeking approval from others. Joseph Campbell summarized the road to health well when he said "Follow your bliss!" By paying close attention to what makes you feel good, choosing to focus on and do only these things, while also getting the medical treatment you need, you will dramatically speed your recovery.

Getting from where you are to where you want to be is easier with the right guidance, however. Dr. Friedberg has taken on the important task of showing you how you can treat the psychological components of these illnesses practically and effectively and offers wise advice and tools that can help you take control of your life and health. Prepare to be empowered.

Love and best wishes for a full recovery,
Jacob Teitelbaum, MD

Dr. Teitelbaum is a board certified internist and Medical Director of the Annapolis Center for Effective CFS/Fibromyalgia Therapies (410-266-6958). Having suffered with and overcome these illnesses in 1975, he spent the next 30 years creating, researching, and teaching about effective therapies. He is the senior author of the landmark study "Effective Treatment of Chronic Fatigue Syndrome and Fibromyalgia—a Placebo-controlled Study" and lectures internationally. He is also the author of the best-selling book

"From Fatigued to Fantastic!" , " Three Steps to Happiness! Healing through Joy", and the recently released "Pain Free 1-2-3- A Proven Program to Get YOU Pain Free! " His web site can be found at: www.Vitality101.com.

Preface

This book is primarily written for those who have chronic fatigue syndrome (CFS) or fibromyalgia (FM). However, even without a formal diagnosis, this book may be helpful to you if, in the past six months or more, you've either been tired most of the time or experienced general bodily pain. Check the list below to see if you also have one or more of the following eight specific symptoms (these symptoms are characteristic of CFS but commonly occur in FM as well):

- Post-exertional malaise (feeling worse after physical or mental exertion)

- Muscle pain in your legs, arms, neck, and/or back

- Joint pain in your knees, shoulders, wrists, and/or elbows

- Memory or concentration difficulty

- Unrefreshing sleep (i.e., waking up feeling tired)

- Headaches that occur or worsen when you are more fatigued

■   Sore throats (apart from colds or flu)

■   Tender or sore lymph glands in your neck or armpits, (apart from colds or flu)

A formal diagnosis of CFS requires four out of these eight symptoms. However, if you have persistent fatigue or pain and only one of these symptoms, this book may still be helpful to you.

Of course, it's important to see your doctor first to determine if any identifiable medical conditions, such as anemia or thyroid deficiency, are present. These conditions may well improve with medications. On the other hand, if your doctor cannot find a medical condition that fully explains your fatigue or pain, then you may have CFS or FM or something similar.

Only a very small number of doctors—those who understand these illnesses—will make a diagnosis of CFS or FM. Usually, even if you're reporting characteristic symptoms of CFS or FM, you'll be told that you're okay or healthy and don't have a serious disease. This does little to address what you can do to help yourself—but that's what this book offers: a user-friendly path to improvement designed for people with persistent fatigue or pain.

PART I

Definitions, Possible Causes, and Lifestyle Factors

The chapters in part I explore definitions, possible causes, and lifestyle factors in chronic fatigue syndrome (CFS) and fibromyalgia (FM). Chapter 1 defines both illnesses clearly and simply; chapter 2 explores various possible causes. Chapter 3 explains why both you and your doctor will benefit from viewing these conditions as mind-body ailments. Chapter 4 sets up the critical premise that personality traits and lifestyle factors play an important role in the development and persistence of CFS and FM. Chapter 5 chronicles how these personality factors profoundly affected the course of my own CFS illness. Chapter 6 reveals how the impact and severity of these illnesses are influenced by "mind" factors—particularly by coping skills that you can learn in order to positively control these difficult conditions.

CHAPTER 1

Defining CFS and FM: Getting It Right

CFS and FM are grouped together in this book because they share a number of perplexing characteristics that baffle both sufferers and their health care providers. For example, some individuals show dramatic and unpredictable fluctuations in their symptoms; they may function almost normally one day only to collapse into bed the next. About one in three affected individuals can work full-time, but many others are disabled from work or even homebound. Laura Hillenbrand, author of the best-selling *Seabiscuit*, is an individual with a severe case of CFS; she dictated her book while lying flat on her back in bed with her eyes closed.

Yet people who are severely ill may still have brief periods when they can do a lot more. On the other hand, higher functioning individuals who are less severely ill may suddenly crash and be unable to carry out their usual responsibilities for weeks or even months. Sometimes unexpected, long-term improvements occur—only to be followed by prolonged relapses. Additionally, CFS and FM share many symptoms, including persistent, unusual fatigue, flu-like symptoms, widespread pain, sleep disturbance, and cognitive difficulties. Fatigue symptoms are more prominent in CFS, while pain symptoms are more common in FM.

We don't know yet what causes CFS or FM. Without laboratory tests, diagnoses are largely based on patient-reported symptoms. Skeptics point out that some studies of these illnesses reveal high levels of psychiatric disorders among individuals with CFS and FM. Yet, many people with CFS and FM do not have psychiatric disorders. The absence of an accepted medical cause, combined with these high levels of psychiatric disorders, leads many physicians to view these patients as fakers. Medical rejection of CFS has led to public skepticism. FM, given its longer history in medicine, may have somewhat greater credibility.

At this point, neither of these illnesses is medically curable, although drug treatments and—more often—behavioral therapy may help to reduce symptoms, strengthen coping abilities, and improve functioning for some people. In long-term studies, many CFS and FM patients show some level of improvement, but less than 10 percent report complete recovery.

Definition of CFS

The Centers for Disease Control defines chronic fatigue syndrome as at least six months of persistent debilitating fatigue not attributable to any identifiable medical condition (Fukuda et al. 1994). Four out of eight secondary symptoms must also be present. These secondary symptoms are:

- Post-exertional malaise (feeling worse after physical or mental exertion)

- Muscle pain in your legs, arms, neck, and/or back

- Joint pain in your knees, shoulders, wrists, and/or elbows

- Memory or concentration difficulty

- Unrefreshing sleep (i.e., waking up feeling tired)

- Headaches that occur or worsen when you are more fatigued

- Sore throats (apart from colds or flu)

- Tender or sore lymph glands in your neck or armpits (apart from colds or flu)

A large number of people with CFS report a sudden onset of the illness, often within a few days to a few weeks. Based on a major prevalence study (Jason et al. 1999), Leonard Jason, an expert on CFS, and his colleagues estimated that 870,000 people in the U.S. have CFS; seventy percent of these individuals are women (1999). CFS in women is roughly fifteen times more common than lung cancer or breast cancer, and over forty times more common than AIDS. The stereotype of CFS as an illness of white professional women—"yuppie flu"—is factually incorrect: illness prevalence rates are roughly equal in African-Americans and whites, while in Latinos the rate is roughly two times greater than in whites.

Post-Exertional Malaise: A Key Symptom of CFS

A recent study (Jason et al. 2002) found that one key characteristic distinguished almost all individuals with CFS from those experiencing fatigue as a result of emotional problems: markedly high levels of post-exertional malaise. *Post-exertional malaise* refers to the typical symptom flare-ups that occur after exertion, whether mental or physical. In fact, the ME Society of America (ME stands for myalgic encephalomyelitis, roughly equivalent to CFS) describes CFS/ME specifically as a disease of exercise or exertion intolerance, and believes that the emphasis on the symptom of fatigue is misplaced.

Exertion produces a number of symptoms, but it is the exertion intolerance itself which is the defining feature of the illness, not simply fatigue. Exertion triggers a variety of symptoms in addition to fatigue, including fevers, sore throats, soreness in lymph glands, chills, body aches, muscle weakness, muscle pain, nausea, vomiting, vertigo, cognitive impairments, confusion, and various other symptoms and disturbances. Focusing on exertion intolerance offers a more accurate definition of CFS/ME, and at the same time de-emphasizes the over-broad term "fatigue," which tends to trivialize the illness.

The symptom flare-ups that define post-exertional malaise typically last anywhere from one to twenty-four hours; if particularly severe, they can last for up to two weeks. This is one of the most frustrating symptoms of the illness: whenever you try to do more, to get back to normal, you hit a wall of worsened symptoms.

Definition of FM

Fibromyalgia syndrome is a chronic pain disorder of at least three months' duration. Patients with FM experience widespread pain both above and below the waist and also have CFS-like symptoms, including fatigue, poor sleep, and intense muscle aching and stiffness. But people with FM also have something else: severe pain at multiple sites called *tender points*. A physical examination is necessary to identify these tender points. A sizeable minority of patients also report menstrual difficulties, irritable bowel syndrome, tension, migraine headaches, and Raynaud's disease. The majority say their illness began suddenly. According to the most recent prevalence study (Wolfe et al. 1990), roughly three to six million people in the U.S. have FM; 90 percent are women.

The Change the Name Debate: CFS vs. FM

Apart from the difficulties in defining these illnesses, many activists in the chronic fatigue community—as well as a few sympathetic health care professionals—advocate abandonment of the term "chronic fatigue syndrome." They believe that the name trivializes the illness—anyone can experience fatigue or chronic fatigue from time to time. The much more serious condition of CFS can become confused with this "normal" experience of fatigue. Many of you may have had doctors, family, or friends compare their occasional fatigue to your CFS fatigue. They may not intend to demean your illness, but just making these comparisons shows how very little they understand about the fatigue you experience. Thus, I would agree that the name "chronic fatigue syndrome" doesn't help to advance the illness's credibility.

A "change the name" meeting was held at the 2001 conference of the American Association for Chronic Fatigue Syndrome in Seattle. One alternative considered was "myalgic encephalomyelitis" (ME), the name used in Canada, Europe, and Australia for CFS. A number of other medical-sounding names were also introduced (although some physicians on the name-change panel opposed names based on obscure Greek and Latin words). Other alternatives considered included direct references to neuroendocrine or immune factors—factors believed to play a role in causing CFS.

Although a name change might reduce trivialization and increase credibility, a new name wouldn't change the fact that a CFS diagnosis is based on a collection of symptoms whose causes are unknown. Generally, physicians are uncomfortable seeing patients with vague illnesses—not so much because of the diagnostic label, but because they do not know what to do with them. You need only to look at FM to see how true this is. Despite the medical-sounding name, FM is still considered by many physicians to be a non-illness, unworthy of serious attention.

Some people with CFS believe that their doctors will take them more seriously if their illness is renamed. A CFS patient on an Internet site pointed out that when she told her doctor that she had ME, he took her complaints much more seriously. This person was very excited about this unexpected level of physician support. The real test is always the doctor's willingness to offer hope and help in the process of ongoing care. A name change alone will not accomplish this. Yes, it may change the initial reaction of the physician, but impressive-sounding diagnoses don't guarantee higher credibility or better care. Moreover, if you're depending on the medical establishment to legitimize your illness, you most likely have a long and arduous wait ahead of you.

What is really needed is physician education about the reality of these illnesses as well as solid, innovative research into causes and treatment. Changing the name may offer some benefits, but it's not nearly as important.

Differences Between CFS and FM

There are few substantive differences between FM and CFS. Although people with CFS tend to report more fatigue and those with FM tend to report more pain, fatigue and pain are often present in both illnesses. Indeed, about one out of three people with CFS also has diagnosable FM.

FM symptoms may be more treatable with medication, given that pain treatment is better established than fatigue treatment. However, medical review studies (see chapter 18) suggest that many people with FM—as well as many with CFS—do not substantially benefit from medical treatments. More optimistically, behavioral treatments—like those described in this book—can benefit one-half to two-thirds of people with these illnesses.

CHAPTER 2

The Ongoing Search for Causes

Scores of scientific hypotheses have been proposed to explain CFS and FM. Some medical theories focus on immune system defects, some on stress hormones, and some on viral infections, while still others reduce CFS and FM to psychological disorders. A number of false starts in both CFS and FM research have generated excitement about possible causes and treatments; however, early positive reports have often led to disappointment when later studies failed to support them. I'm very cautious about any theory until there's firm and convincing evidence for it. All of the theories below either have strong supporting evidence or focus specifically on aspects of CFS and FM that seem especially important. (An additional neuroendocrine theory of CFS, based on abnormalities in the stress hormone cortisol, is discussed in chapter 4.)

Immune Defects

The often reported flu-like symptoms of these two illnesses have led scientists to a search for an underlying viral or bacterial cause. However, no specific bug—including Epstein-Barr virus, cytomegalovirus, and human herpesvirus 6—has consistently been linked with either illness. Lacking a disease-creating bug, researchers have focused instead on possible defects in the immune system.

Immune defects can produce abnormally high levels of disease-fighting cells or substances in the body. These disease-fighting entities cause the flu-like symptoms that you normally get when you have a cold or flu. However, according to this theory, in CFS and FM, you get the flu symptoms from the immune defect itself, without a triggering virus or bacterium.

A potentially promising immune marker in CFS is called upregulated *RNase L*. RNase L is one of the immune system's key disease-fighting enzymes. It breaks down invading viruses and destroys infected cells. The *RNase L pathway* refers to a sequence of chemical changes that takes place in your white blood cells when you are fighting off a viral infection. This chemical process has all sorts of effects at a microscopic level which could well lead to many of the symptoms CFS patients complain about.

In studies conducted by Robert Suhadolnik and his colleagues at the Temple University School of Medicine in Philadelphia (1999), higher than normal levels of RNase L have consistently been found in CFS patients. Moreover, RNase L overactivity has been correlated with a lower state of general health in CFS patients and illness improvements have been associated with the return of the RNase L activity level to normal. Kenny De Meirleir of the Fatigue Clinic in Brussels, Belgium and colleagues have also found evidence that the RNase L enzyme is only half its normal molecular weight in CFS patients (2000). Further replication of these promising results may get us closer to identifying a biological marker for CFS.

Sleep Disturbance

Sleep disturbance is an almost universal complaint in CFS and FM; sleep disorders in these illnesses have been documented in a number of sleep studies. According to Ian Hickie and Tracy Davenport (1999) and Harvey Moldofsky (1993), CFS and FM are best viewed as disorders of the sleep-wake cycle. The actual sleep disturbance itself involves a reduction in deep (slow wave) sleep—a type of sleep which is essential for a good night's restorative slumber. These researchers have proposed that these abnormal sleep patterns in CFS and FM cause two major disturbances: one in the sleep-wake rhythms and the other in cortisol, melatonin, and serotonin (hormones that normally help to regulate the sleep-wake cycle). As a result, people with CFS and FM are in a half-asleep zombie-like state during their waking hours—and partially awake and restless during their sleeping hours.

The evidence for this theory is stronger for FM patients, who consistently show a disturbance of deep sleep. Indeed, in an interesting related finding, healthy individuals who were deprived of deep sleep for several days developed an FM-like illness (Moldofsky et al. 1975).

The next step in advancing this theory would involve sleep treatment studies using behavioral methods or medication—preferably both. In fact, behavioral treatment studies in CFS suggest that sleep can be improved with good sleep hygiene (see chapter 8). If this theory is correct, then effective treatment of sleep disturbance may lead to major improvements in these illnesses.

Is Trauma Related to Illness Development?

Lifestyle stress—in combination with a single overpowering traumatic event—can help to trigger CFS and FM. The two scientific studies below shed light on how this can happen.

CFS and Trauma

In a Swedish study conducted by Tores Theorell and his colleagues (1999), a group of forty-six people with CFS who experienced stressful events just prior to illness onset were compared with a control group of healthy people who experienced stressful events at about the same time. There was a dramatic rise in fatigue in both groups during the peak three-month period surrounding the stressful events. However, the CFS group reported a greater incidence of marital separations and increased responsibility at work as major stressors—and these events weren't simply confined to the months just before CFS began, but were distributed over the entire year preceding onset of CFS. This suggests that stressful life events can lead to persistent fatigue—and for some individuals, significant illness may be the result.

This same study also found that the number of infections and fatigue symptoms in CFS patients increased during the year before the dramatic rise in fatigue. It's possible that these infections made the people who became ill more vulnerable to the negative life events that occurred. (Correlations between stressful events and infections in healthy adults have been established in previous studies—e.g., Cohen 2005.) A number of other studies in CFS also implicate pre-illness stress as a triggering factor.

Not only can stress and trauma precede these illnesses, the sudden onset of these disabling conditions can trigger trauma-like feelings. Trauma symptoms may include nightmares, forceful avoidance of thoughts or activities associated with the traumatic event, increased agitation, insomnia, and excessive attention to what is going on internally within your body as well as around you. Trauma-like symptoms can also be a reaction to an increased sensitivity to stress—day-to-day stressors that you may have previously tolerated without adverse effects may now become disruptive.

FM and Trauma

Jeffrey Sherman and his colleagues evaluated ninety-three patients with FM for trauma symptoms (2000). Fifty-six percent of this sample reported significant levels of trauma symptoms. Patients with trauma symptoms also had greater levels of pain, emotional distress, life interference, and disability than those patients with FM who didn't have trauma symptoms. So, not only do many people with FM have to deal with FM symptoms, they also have additional emotional symptoms that can make the entire FM experience that much worse.

■ Beth's Story: Trauma in a Person with FM

At thirty-eight, Beth had suffered from FM for ten years, but was able to continue working as a library assistant at a local high school. During the final year of her employment, a new authoritarian boss took over and began to treat her with condescension and arrogance. Beth was disturbed by this change but she continued with her job. However, when Beth attempted to keep a student out of the library during a final exam, the new library head physically pushed her away from the student, admonishing her that she shouldn't do that. Beth was emotionally devastated and became quite sick after this event; she began to experience high levels of anxiety, increased sleep disturbance, and cognitive difficulties. Despite a love for the job she'd held for many years, she could no longer work; she took a medical leave.

Beth's FM may well have increased her vulnerability to the emotional damage of the pushing incident. Eventually, stress reduction exercises and the support provided by an FM group lessened Beth's emotional and physical symptoms, and she began working as a volunteer for the elderly.

Despite the negative impact of trauma symptoms, they can often be successfully treated by using the relaxation, stress reduction, and lifestyle change techniques described in this book. (Of course, if the trauma symptoms are stubbornly persistent and debilitating, professional help is in order.)

CHAPTER 3

Why Mind-Body Dualism Doesn't Help

I believe that CFS and FM have both physical and psychological causes, so it's counterproductive to reduce them to just one or the other. However, because many in the medical community view these conditions as non-illnesses, people with CFS and FM may become very defensive whenever anyone suggests that psychological factors play any role in CFS or FM. Yet you may be more receptive to physicians or other health professionals who talk about stress factors if they are sensitive to—rather than dismissive of—your illness concerns; and of course, if they offer potential help.

The Ongoing Mind-Body Battles

CFS and FM patients—as well as a handful of sympathetic health professionals—often feel pitted against a much larger group of health care practitioners and medical researchers who reject these illnesses. For instance, whenever a new study suggests psychological causation, an equal and opposite reaction develops in CFS/FM activists: they vigorously dispute and dismiss the findings.

One of the more articulate critics of psychological causation in CFS is British psychologist Ellen Goudsmit. Goudsmit has effectively challenged the findings of many published articles that implicate psychological factors in these illnesses. Although many of her arguments are well-reasoned, she is also beholden to a rigid mind-body dualism—so much so that I suspect she would *never* support a role for psychological factors in CFS, no matter what the evidence.

The underlying problem is an unyielding mind-body dualism— from all sides. It seems that you can only be in one camp or the other, not both.

Mind-Body Dualism and the ME Society of America

This mind-body split is also embodied in the founding principles of the ME Society of America. (ME, or myalgic encephalomyelitis, is the term used for CFS in Canada, Europe, and Australia.) These principles state that ME (or CFS) is a true medical condition validated by numerous studies showing various biological disturbances (e.g., neurally mediated hypotension, a blood pressure abnormality). According to this society, these medical problems explain, for instance, why patients are sometimes bedridden. They also cite a variety of other physiological abnormalities and agents as related to ME, including muscle myopathy, elevated lactic acid in the muscles, viruses, bacteria, immune system dysregulation, and neuroendocrine abnormalities.

Although it's true that findings of these physiological abnormalities and agents in CFS/ME have been published, it's not accurate to say that these abnormalities fully explain CFS/ME symptoms. Indeed, to make this statement is an unscientific leap from inconsistent results and unproven theories—an act which reflects, in my view, a somewhat desperate attempt to advance the science well beyond the data that is available; this detracts from the credibility of CFS/ME rather than advancing it.

In addition, the ME Society's founding principles reject all behavioral and stress reduction treatments for CFS/ME. In their view, any behavioral intervention that works—to whatever degree—means that the individual who benefited from it cannot actually have CFS/ME. This reflects yet again the wearying mind-body split in both medicine and our culture in general. The Society's underlying premise is that CFS/ME must have a biomedical basis and therefore must be treated medically. So any individual with CFS/ME whose illness has improved from lifestyle changes is persona non grata—a strangely invalidating premise for an organization that seeks to heighten credibility of this illness and provide accurate information about it!

The Downside of "Biology Is Everything"

If you view treatment of these illnesses as a search for purely biological causes, then you're ignoring what may be most helpful to you right now: the control that you can exert over your own beliefs, personal stress levels, and activities.

When I was in that biology-is-everything camp, I sustained myself with the belief that I would find a practitioner who could cure me—but after eighteen years of slavish adherence to the biological model, I had little to show for it other than a depleted bank account. Now, I don't intend to dismiss medical and alternative treatments totally: a small number have indeed been shown to be helpful. If you view these treatments as part of a personal effort at improving illness management rather than as an answer, a cure, or salvation, then you're much more likely to attain some benefit.

Why I Left the Mind-Body Debate

Until a few years ago, I would have wholeheartedly agreed with the ME Society of America; I, too, believed in the pure biological model. But over the past several years I've learned two important things that have changed my rigid view of these illnesses: First, finding a cure could occur well after my lifetime, and I'm not willing to just wait. Second, I can substantially improve my illness—if not fully recover—through lifestyle adjustments and stress reduction techniques.

Why would anyone argue against self-controlling these illnesses if it can be achieved?

Do People with CFS and FM View Stress as an Important Illness Factor?

I can understand why people with these illnesses don't want to high-light the role of stress. Acknowledging stress as a factor in your illness to doctors, family, and friends may seem risky—they may think that even you believe psychological factors cause CFS and FM. But you can still legitimately view your illness as having multiple causes. In a study of 258 CFS patients that I conducted with Lucy Dechene, Maggie McKenzie, and Robert Fontanetta (2000), we asked participants to rate a number of factors as "important" or "not important" causes of their illness. Roughly 90 percent rated immune/viral factors as most impor-tant, with 63 percent rating persistent stress as the second most important causal factor. (Other factors rated as important included genetic and hereditary influence, diet, and emotional trauma.) Thus, CFS patients themselves acknowledge the role of stress in their illness, even though they don't necessarily rate it as the primary cause.

Interestingly, the patients in this study who said their illnesses were improving were more likely to rate stress as an important cause (as compared to those with worsening illness). It's possible that for the improving group, stress was simply a more important cause. However, in my experience, the ability to recognize persistent stress and then take affirmative steps to reduce that stress is a crucial element in getting on an improvement track.

Mind-Body Linkages: Behavioral Change Can Trigger Physiological Change

At the January 2001 meeting of the American Association for Chronic Fatigue Syndrome, a research scientist presented data on altered immune function in CFS and the possibilities of correcting the abnor-mality; the audience was very impressed. However, when one ques-tioner asked about using stress reduction techniques to improve immune function in CFS, the members of the audience murmured in disapproval; the speaker concurred, saying, "This is an organic illness, we need organic treatments." But this is simply not true. Changing behavior, whether it is part of the formal treatment or not, can improve your physiological functioning—and such improvements may well lead to illness reduction.

The linkage between behavior, immune function, and illness is far from proven in CFS and FM. However, a recent CFS behavioral treatment study in England (Cleary 2002) found that those patients who improved had healthier levels of cortisol at the end of treatment. (Low cortisol levels and immune dysfunction may play a role in CFS—see chapter 4.) This is the first CFS study to show how behavioral change can lead to physiological improvements.

How Lifestyle and Attitude Impact Chronic Conditions

The concept of mind-body integration in disease has only recently begun to penetrate Western medicine. A landmark article by George Engel in *Science* (1977) suggested that all illnesses involve an interaction of physical, mental, behavioral, and social factors. Reducing illness and disease only to physical factors ignores the major impact of your personal behavior on your illness condition. For people with CFS and FM, this means that illness effects on your life depend not only on the physical disease process itself (whatever that may be), but just as importantly on your attitude toward them.

Lifestyle factors have been shown to be important determinants of many so-called organic illnesses. It's now common knowledge that diet is related to the risk of heart disease and certain cancers. More recently, emotional factors such as anger have also been implicated in heart disease (Ketterer, Mahr, and Goldberg 2000), while bottling up emotions appears to be related to certain cancers (Garssen 2004). By extending this logic to treatment strategies, dietary change and stress reduction may lessen the risks of getting these illnesses and improve your potential outcome once you have them.

You definitely won't hear advocates for chronic conditions such as heart disease and cancer denying the importance of lifestyle change and stress reduction. Not only do these factors help in managing these illnesses, but in many cases, they actually lead to improvements as well. Of course, these conditions have a level of medical credibility that makes it easier for patients to accept the potential benefits of behavior and lifestyle change. But the principle is the same: if behavioral methods can offer significant benefit, why not use them?

Even if you assume that effective medical intervention will arrive one day, lifestyle management techniques will still remain important. Heart disease provides a good parallel: effective medications and surgeries are available for the disease; however, long-term management of the disease depends on lifestyle factors such as good social support, stress management, diet, and exercise. And these behavioral factors haven't simply fallen away because we now have better medical treatment than we once did.

Controlling CFS and FM Through Lifestyle Change

As with other chronic illnesses, understanding mind-body interactions is important to understanding CFS and FM. Without the support of a healthy lifestyle, potentially effective treatments become far less effective. Even with medical advances, it's most unlikely that you'll ever be able to simply graft your hustle-bustle pre-illness lifestyle onto a new improved self.

Although I used to view any limitation as a cause for pessimism, I can now turn the half-empty glass around and fill it with the good results I have achieved. I do this by challenging my old negative assumptions and redefining what is important and necessary to have a good quality of life.

By fostering improvements through your own personal efforts, you become far less dependent on questionable medical and alternative approaches. By taking control of your illness you have less need to prove to physicians—or anyone else for that matter—that you are, indeed, ill. For many people with CFS and FM, this may also result in a decreased dependence on incomplete and unproven theories of illness causation.

Effective Drug Treatment of Migraines; Why Lifestyle Is Still Important

There are a number of similarities between people who suffer from persistent and severe migraines and those with CFS and FM. Both conditions can cause disability, cognitive difficulties, social restrictions, and exercise intolerance. Fortunately for many migraine sufferers, so-called triptan-type drugs (e.g., Imitrex) can avert migraine headaches at an early stage. For those individuals with occasional migraines—say two times a month—triptan drugs are sufficiently effective to provide relief and avoid sick days and other limitations.

But for those who have frequent, severe migraines, Imitrex and other headache drugs can prove problematic: regular use of them can cause dependence, rebound headaches when the drug effect wears off, and a loss of effectiveness of the drug over time. Severe migraine sufferers also tend to be uncomfortable with the frequent use of headache drugs and would prefer not to use them; they want to avoid the problems of dependence, side effects, and withdrawal—as well as the high cost.

In several studies of migraine sufferers (Holm et al. 1997; Spierings et al. 2001; Wacogne et al. 2003), stress has been found to be a headache trigger. For those who are willing to acknowledge a role for stress and seek help in managing it, reductions in migraine frequency, severity, and duration are possible.

The Present and the Future

I respect anyone's desire to pursue the medication route for their illness. But if you pursue that route to the complete exclusion of lifestyle change, your potential improvement will necessarily be limited. One day, medical research will have more to offer you than it does now. Unfortunately, in the case of CFS and FM, there is little in the way of reliable drug (or other medical) interventions. And an endless pursuit of questionable, often expensive, and sometimes high-risk remedies isn't the answer. This is a conclusion I reached after eighteen years of illness—and my conviction grows ever stronger with my increasing ability to control my illness without treatment.

CHAPTER 4

Helping and Hard Driving: How This Personality Style Can Hurt You

Do you have helping and hard-driving traits? Take this short yes-or-no quiz to find out:

1. I often overdo my activities and use up my energy.

2. I must keep busy at all times.

3. I have trouble expressing anger.

4. Relaxing is difficult for me.

5. It is essential that others view me as a nice person.

6. I receive little emotional support from others.

If you answered yes to at least three items, including 1 or 2, 3 or 4, and 5 or 6, then you probably have helping and hard-driving personality traits. Items 1 and 2 capture the hard-driving, nonstop activity that describes many people with CFS and FM. Items 3 and 4 target the common inability to relax mentally and emotionally. Items 5 and 6 identify beliefs related to helping and receiving help from others that in their extreme forms can lead to exhaustion and pain. The importance of these ideas is explained throughout the book.

What Does "Helping and Hard Driving" Mean?

"Helping and hard driving" refers to the overextended lifestyles of people with CFS or FM. They are often working full-time, taking care of families and helping others—and then squeezing even more activities, such as volunteer work and exercise programs, into their remaining hours. People with CFS and FM also tend to be highly responsible, conscientious, and caretaking of others (particularly in FM). Yet they often feel inadequate for failing to meet the high standards they set for themselves, both before and after the onset of their illness. Overdoing to the point of collapse is commonplace. *These helping and hard-driving personality traits play an important role in the onset and persistence of these illnesses.*

Despite these feelings of inadequacy, many people with CFS and FM will say that they were quite happy with their lives before they became ill. That may be; however, many individuals also led unhealthy, overextended lifestyles before illness onset. When you were well, you probably did a lot to achieve certain things and allowed little time for recuperation and personal reflection; you may have ignored the effects of your busy lifestyle on your health and well-being. Although now you may be hypersensitive to stress, you were probably blind to the stress already in your life before you became ill.

Even after the illness begins, your lifestyle may still be overextended—although probably to a lesser degree, and not just in terms of paid employment. You could be spreading yourself too thin with too many commitments. Even if you are quite limited and now do much less than you did when you were well, you may quickly use up what energy you have in your attempts to get back on your old fast track.

More generally, your helping others may be motivated, in part, by your desire to be viewed as a nice or good person. Or, you may be seeking love, approval, and support from people who aren't capable of giving it—or less capable than you'd like. This amounts to pursuing life goals that are mostly or entirely unattainable, and results in endless frustration, exhaustion, and more stress. When energy is higher, these hyperactive traits push individuals to the extremes of overwork; when energy is depleted, these traits propel individuals to inevitable collapse. This overwork-collapse cycle is then perpetuated by ever more desperate attempts to maintain an impossibly high level of functioning.

Evidence for the Helping and Hard-Driving Lifestyle

When Harvard sociologist Norma Ware conducted in-depth interviews of fifty CFS patients to evaluate their lifestyles both before and after they became ill (1993), she found that these individuals had been strongly committed both to work and family caregiving. CFS sufferers described themselves as living overcommitted and overextended lives, as well as having a tendency to place the interests of others before their own. The results of the study suggest that those who developed the illness were exhausted from their overcommitted lifestyles well before they became ill. Perhaps surprisingly, 44 percent of interviewed patients indicated that the illness actually led to positive changes in their life priorities. These changes included both greater attention to self-care and a decreased emphasis on work and caregiving.

A later personality study done by psychologist Boudewijn Van Houdenhouve and colleagues (1995) found that individuals with CFS and FM were significantly more *action-prone* prior to becoming ill, in comparison to patients with other chronic conditions or psychiatric disorders. (An individual who is highly action-prone is passionate, strong-willed, energetic, and driven.) The CFS and FM patients in this study were likely to agree with statements such as: "I have always been an active and busy person," "I do not like to postpone things," and "I love making a supreme effort."

A more recent study (2001) by this same research group not only replicated these findings on a second CFS and FM sample, but also found that the spouses of these patients also rated them as action-prone. This is an important validation of the earlier findings—

particularly since those earlier findings had been dismissed by skeptics who suggested that people with CFS and FM had simply exaggerated their pre-illness activity levels.

A similar study authored by Suzan Lewis and her colleagues (1994) compared subjects with CFS, subjects with irritable bowel syndrome, and healthy control subjects on their levels of achievement motivation. Lewis found no differences between the two illness groups in type A behavior (a high achievement personality trait). However, both illness groups rated themselves as more hard-driving prior to becoming ill than healthy controls did. The CFS group also rated themselves as better listeners than the other two groups.

These studies suggest that people who develop CFS or FM often have led highly stressful, overactive lifestyles without regard to its effects on their personal health. Persistently high activity levels can overburden the body with too many physical and emotional demands—and these stressful demands can trigger physical collapse and illness. (This may be especially true for those with childhood victimization experiences; often these individuals will overwork themselves in order to maintain self-esteem and divert attention from feelings of anxiety and depression.)

The Helping and Hard-Driving Lifestyle and Its Effects on Stress Hormones

According to Christine Heim, a biopsychologist at the Centers for Disease Control, and her colleagues (Heim, Ehlert, and Hellhammer 2000), persistently high levels of physical or mental stress may, in susceptible individuals, lead to abnormally low levels of cortisol, a stress-related hormone. In turn, low levels of cortisol may trigger various stress-related disorders, such as CFS and FM.

Low cortisol levels have been found in people with CFS and FM as well as in other stressed groups (e.g., overtrained athletes, overworked laborers, and teachers suffering from burnout). This suggests that for some individuals there's an abnormality in the body's response to stress. People with CFS and FM are more reactive to a wide range of stressors, including loud noises, bright lights, medication, odors, chemicals, and mentally challenging tasks. For instance, in one study (Wood et al. 1994), people with CFS showed greater physical and psychological reactions while performing mental arithmetic than healthy subjects and psychiatric controls.

What is the role of cortisol in our physiological functioning? Let's focus on its relation to immune functioning. Healthy levels of cortisol protect the body's immune system and help keep it in check. Low levels of cortisol allow the immune system to go into overdrive, as if mounting a defense against an invading virus or harmful bacteria. This immune activation process may trigger fatigue-related symptoms and exhaustion—symptoms that you'd normally only get if you had a cold or flu. (This may explain the flu-like symptoms of CFS and FM, which can occur even when no virus or bacterium can be detected.) Heim and her colleagues believe that low cortisol may also play an important role in the development of other immune-related illnesses, including autoimmune disorders, allergies, and asthma.

Given this relationship in CFS and FM between chronic stress, cortisol, and the immune system, lifestyle changes that significantly reduce stress may help to:

■ restore healthy levels of cortisol

■ dampen an overactive immune system

■ lessen fatigue and flu-like symptoms

In fact, a recent behavioral treatment study not yet published (Cleary 2002) found that those CFS patients who improved with treatment also had elevated (healthier) levels of cortisol compared to their pretreatment levels. (Behavioral treatment involves lifestyle changes and stress reduction techniques—the types of improvement tools offered in this book.)

Why Focus on Personality Factors?

Many people with CFS and FM are reluctant to consider personality factors, perhaps fearing that such an emphasis would reduce the credibility of these illnesses. After all, if personality traits are only a single factor in the mix of physical and psychological ingredients that cause CFS and FM, shouldn't the focus be on identifying biomedical factors? I understand these concerns; in no way do I wish to discourage medical research into causes and potentially effective treatments—I'm simply looking at the aspects of these illnesses that you can do something about right now.

Linking personality and stress to illness severity in CFS and FM is not meant to negate the powerful role of biological factors in any way. The role of cortisol in immune function, as explained above, suggests how stress may lead to a variety of immune-related disorders, including CFS and FM. Unfortunately, effective treatment of the biomedical factors in these illnesses is not yet available. But effective treatment of behavioral, psychological, personality, and stress factors is available— not as a cure, but as a vehicle to greatly improved quality of life and lessened illness severity.

CHAPTER 5

My CFS Experience: How Life Balance Leads to Major Improvements

I've had CFS now for twenty-five years. It began suddenly, while I was jogging my usual five miles around the Central Park reservoir in New York City. Pressure headaches and fatigue increased over a three-week period until I felt so exhausted that I couldn't continue my daily running schedule.

Over the next several years, I visited every sort of doctor—from internists to neurologists to sports medicine specialists. No one could explain my unusual symptoms (pressure headaches, mental confusion, constant fatigue, and the inability to exercise). Finally, in the late 1980s, I read the definition of CFS in a medical journal and I recognized my symptoms and felt some sense of relief. I was not alone, this was a medical condition.

Now that I knew what I had, my next step was to get well. I had no interest in coping with this illness, I just wanted to be well—and nothing short of that goal was acceptable. I knew I couldn't be happy as long as I was ill. If I continued to have symptoms, my life was not just limited, it was unbearable. As a result, I felt depressed, frustrated, and angry—both with my clueless doctors and with my own inability to help myself.

Although I had to give up exercise, even in small doses, I could still work as a clinical psychologist. Of course this ability to continue work was important, but I didn't really appreciate it. It was all or nothing for me. My quality of life suffered, not only because of the illness itself, but also because of my intolerance of it. (Many people with these illnesses are stuck, to varying degrees, with these understandable but very damaging attitudes. After all, why would anyone want to put up with a debilitating illness if there were any possible way to get well?)

Eventually I realized that a medical diagnosis didn't necessarily lead to an effective treatment or cure. Over the years, my illness slowly worsened. All of my efforts to halt the slide, much less improve or recover, worked temporarily at best.

How CFS and FM May Begin and Worsen

Many people with CFS and FM, though not all, experienced a rapid onset of their illness; some describe it as "hitting like a bolt of lightning." A sudden, debilitating illness can be a shocking and sometimes traumatizing event. Without someone to make sense of it, such as a physician, the confusion and stress can be even greater.

At first, you may try to ignore the symptoms and press on with your usual activities. If you are able to pass for healthy by doing what you normally do, you may feel you have achieved something, despite the illness. Yet you may have lost the good feelings that you had before the illness set in. If your efforts to press on falter, you may then be forced to cut back on your active lifestyle. Doing much less than you want is demoralizing; sometimes you may feel like giving up in despair.

My case of CFS was relatively mild. Perhaps this is because my unhealthy behaviors weren't the kind that exhaust people to the point where they end up in bed: I didn't have the usual workaholic or sacrifice-for-others philosophy that many people with CFS and FM have.

Instead, my major unhealthy behavior was a self-imposed social isolation. This lack of healthy relationships seems to have been an important triggering factor in my CFS. Also, my illness worsened gradually over time. This occurred, I believe, for two reasons: first, I did little to remedy my lack of social relationships; and second, I added to my lifestyle another illness-worsening behavior—choosing to work longer and longer hours. For several years I became almost totally work-focused. I viewed recreation as a waste of time and I stressed myself further by feeling contempt for anyone who didn't work as much as I did.

Despite my worsening illness, I maintained a hectic lifestyle of fifty-hour work weeks. I was single-mindedly focused on professional accomplishment, almost to the exclusion of anything else. Over a five-year period in the 1990s, I brought work with me on every single vacation. But still, I didn't correlate my behavior with my illness. Because CFS (and FM) symptoms are so physical and so unlike familiar stress reactions such as anxiety and depression, I failed to make the connection between my lifestyle and my illness.

Symptoms and Vacations: Why Illness May Improve in a Different Environment

The main reason why I was confused about my illness during the first few years had to do with the dramatic improvement I experienced whenever I left New York City for week-long vacations—or even just weekend visits to my family in rural upstate New York. I could understand feeling less pressure and more relaxed when I left my work behind, but I also felt much less ill. My symptoms disappeared almost entirely, especially in the beginning stages of my illness. At the time, I attributed these improvements to cleaner air rather than to the effect of a relaxing friendly social environment. (And this made a certain amount of sense; I had been tested for chemical sensitivities and found to be highly sensitive to auto exhaust, a persistent problem in traffic-congested New York City.) Because my symptoms were so physical and strange—especially the exercise intolerance—I didn't realize how they could be, at least in part, a reflection of my lifestyle.

Fatigue in CFS and FM is quite different from normal fatigue and may be experienced as flu-like symptoms, brain fog, wired feelings, or a heavy "molasses-like" sensation throughout the body. Given my clearly abnormal type of fatigue, it made sense to me to look for environmental factors—e.g., toxic chemicals and allergens—to explain my symptoms and their abrupt disappearance whenever I was away from New York City. Perhaps some would say I was in denial about the importance of psychological factors in my illness. If a mental health professional could have explained to me how social isolation and overwork affected my illness, I would have tried to do something about it. When I did speak to a psychologist about my illness, she made some good observations about my lifestyle (apart from the illness), but she never put together a usable improvement plan that I could try. (Unfortunately, many mental health professionals are either skeptical of CFS and FM or do not know how to identify mind-body connections in these perplexing conditions.)

I decided to move from New York City to a cleaner and less chemically toxic environment, and relocated to a suburban area of eastern Long Island where I had felt good on previous vacations. However, my symptoms persisted. I was perplexed, annoyed, and fed up. Perhaps another move would help? When I was at a sports camp in rural Connecticut, my illness would again disappear, almost entirely. I decided to move to that area of Connecticut. Once again, I thought this was the clean environment I needed, but my symptoms didn't disappear; in fact, after this second move, they worsened. I felt even more frustrated and demoralized than before.

During this time I underwent a variety of expensive alternative medicine treatments, including oral and IV vitamins, allergy shots, homeopathy, chelation, and special diets. I experienced some improvement but my limitations were still present—I couldn't jog or even walk for exercise.

It took me almost two decades to realize that deliverance from CFS wasn't going to come from outside treatments. I think my stubbornness was due to my low level of impairment: I could do *most* of the things that I wanted, just not all. The less you're impaired, the less incentive you have to reevaluate your life. On the other hand, if you're suddenly crushed by disabling symptoms, your need to reevaluate your life becomes much more urgent.

What Worked for Me: Changing My Environment at Home

About eighteen years into my illness, I decided to start playing two or three recreational volleyball games each week during the summer months. This involved brief bursts of exertion with frequent rest periods in between—exercise I could handle. (I had always found volleyball to be uplifting and symptom-reducing, although this effect never lasted for more than a day.)

During this summer I started to feel better—perhaps 30 to 40 percent better on a daily basis. I had never experienced such an improvement before. During this time, I also cut back on my crushing workload and made time for relationships that were becoming more important to me. As a psychologist myself, I often point out mind-body connections to help other people understand their feelings and symptoms, but until this point I had never made the connection between changing my own lifestyle and feeling better.

That crucial summer was seven years ago. Since then, I've devoted more time to recreation and relationships—and increased my improvement to 50 to 60 percent. At times I've even felt nearly well. I still can't do regular aerobic exercise, but now the malaise that plagued me for years has been replaced by hope and optimism. I don't view my lifestyle changes as a cure (although I certainly wish they could work that well!) If I slip back into overwork and social isolation, I know my symptoms will worsen. Clearly, there is an underlying physical problem that cannot be corrected entirely by behavioral change. But I know from personal experience that behavioral change is very powerful. As you read this book, I ask that you keep an open mind about what you can do to help yourself feel better—perhaps very much better.

Why Minor Lifestyle Changes May Not Work

In my previous book, *Coping With Chronic Fatigue Syndrome: Nine Things You Can Do* (1995), I described a variety of techniques similar to those in this book. In that earlier work, I viewed these techniques simply as illness coping strategies, rather than as actual improvement techniques; as a result I only prescribed them on a relatively modest level.

I now realize that a much greater commitment to these strategies is necessary for improvement. It may be that you already use some of these techniques occasionally and feel that they help with coping but not actual improvement. In response, I would say that you need to meld these strategies into your daily schedule, rather than just use them occasionally. To receive the maximum benefit from these strategies, they must become as important as anything else that you may have to do during your day.

CHAPTER 6

Can Good Coping and Stress Reduction Improve Illness?

The following list shows how illness improvement and worsening relate to stress and coping. Levels 6 to 10 represent illness improvement. Level 10 indicates cure or recovery, either with no future risk of relapse or some very minimal risk of relapse; level 9 indicates either illness remission or a complete absence of symptoms, but for a time-limited period—say six months to two years; level 8, a reduction in symptoms and disability that may or may not be time-limited; level 7, a reduction in overall stress without any improvement in the illness itself; level 6, improvement in coping skills without improvement in the illness itself. Levels 1 to 5 represent the opposite side of the coin, from no change in illness (level 5) to increased stress, poor coping, and a worsened illness condition (levels 4 to 1).

Levels of Illness Change

10.   Recovery or cure

 9.   Illness remission

 8.   Illness improvement

 7.   Reduced stress (no illness improvement)

 6.   Improved coping (no illness improvement)

 5.   No illness change

 4.   Increased stress (no illness worsening)

 3.   Poor coping (no illness worsening)

 2.   Long duration relapses

 1.   Worsened illness

The important question to derive from this scale is: can reduced stress and improved coping in and of themselves lead to illness improvements? In other words, can a 6 or 7 rating lead directly to an 8 or higher? The studies below on coping, stress reduction, and illness control suggest that this can indeed happen. Of course, illness improvement (level 8) may be far short of everyone's ultimate goal of full and sustained recovery (level 10). But in the absence of full recovery, are you receptive to improving your illness by improving your quality of life? Another way of asking the question is: are you willing to accept three-quarters or even half a loaf if the full loaf isn't available right now? If not, are you depending on a particular level of improvement or recovery in order to pronounce your life good or acceptable? If you *must* have full recovery, then you'll limit your potential to improve—and feel better *now*.

Let's look at the lower end of the scale, from levels 4 to 1; level 4 represents increased levels of stress; level 3, poor or ineffective coping; level 2, long bouts of worsened illness that alternate with your usual level of illness; and level 1, a general worsening of illness. You can ask the opposite question for these levels of illness change: can increased stress and poor coping in and of themselves lead directly to a worsening illness? You may already recognize a connection between high stress, poor coping, and illness flare-ups and setbacks. But will these stress and coping factors actually increase illness severity long term? I believe this is very likely.

The evidence cited below supports my view that coping and stress are related to the severity of your illness.

Studies of Good Coping and Illness Improvement

Several studies of coping as it relates to illness severity and improvement have been done with CFS and FM patients. In general, a personal feeling of control over symptoms has been found to consistently predict better functioning.

Susan Lutgendorf and her colleagues conducted a study of coping and relapse in people with CFS who were in the direct path of Hurricane Andrew (1995). They found that an optimistic coping style was associated with resistance to relapse and improved levels of *interleukin*, a chemical messenger of the immune system associated with CFS-like symptoms. This is particularly important because recent evidence from a number of studies (see chapter 2) suggests that people with CFS show impaired immune function.

Similarly, positive feelings of illness control are also important in improving FM. Susan Buckelew and her colleagues found that people with FM who reported greater feelings of illness control even before a coping skills treatment showed more improvements in physical activity by the end of the treatment (1996). In addition, the patients who actually *improved* their sense of illness control showed reductions in their tender point index, disease severity, and pain. These authors suggest that a sense of illness control may thus be a critical factor in the effectiveness of rehabilitation programs for FM.

A previous study by Buckelew and her research group (1995) also showed that higher feelings of illness control were correlated with less pain and less impairment (this important relationship held up even in the most severely ill and was unrelated to both age and length of illness).

Thus, a more severe illness doesn't necessarily mean helplessness and lack of control—even people with severe illness can feel optimistic and in control. Why? Because people can adjust their expectations so that even modest activity and accomplishment can be appreciated and serve as a source of optimism and inspiration. I've witnessed this kind of attitude many times in people with CFS and FM who can no longer work but still have a good quality of life. By maintaining a sense of psychological control, they reduce symptom-intensifying stress and improve their functioning to the greatest extent possible. For some, that may be a modest (but significant) 20 percent or so, but for others it can be much higher—50 percent or more.

Long-Term Studies and Good Coping

These findings about self-control have also been confirmed in long-term studies. In one such study, researchers found that the strongest predictor of improvement in CFS over an eighteen-month period was (again) the patient's sense of control over his or her symptoms (Vercoulen, Swanink, Fennis, et al. 1996). Their analysis suggested that this sense of control actually reduced fatigue severity itself rather than vice versa (reduced fatigue severity leading to a greater sense of control). This sense of control was more strongly correlated to symptom severity than treatment by medical specialists and alternative practitioners. These findings point to both the importance of good coping and to the inadequate level of medical treatment that's currently available for CFS and FM.

Additionally, a one-year study of CFS patients (Ray, Jeffries, and Weir 1997) demonstrated an interesting relationship between a sense of illness control and impairments: patients who believed that their own actions influenced their illness had less impairment one year later—and this was unrelated to both the severity and length of their illness. In addition, a subtle but important difference was found between those who reported more control over their symptoms and those who did not. For those who felt little control over symptoms, the more they attempted to limit activity and avoid stress, the less they were able to do; whereas for those who reported strong feelings of control over symptoms, limiting activity and stress did not increase impairment.

Personal Illness Control

If you have little faith in your ability to control your illness, you may believe that coping itself can't lead to any real or long-term benefit. If you feel victimized by your illness, you may cope with each symptom flare-up simply by reacting to it, without any long-term strategy on how you might take control. With a greater sense of control, accommodating to your illness can, at times, be a healthy and positive strategy. Activity can be moderated (or paced) so that improvements can develop. Increasing a sense of illness control—rather than simply increasing activity—may be the key factor in effective lifestyle treatments for CFS and FM.

How I Found Illness Control

In my case, I increased illness control in two ways: by identifying what activities made me feel better and doing them more, and by reducing (or stopping) activities that made me feel worse. This may sound pretty straightforward on paper, but putting it into practice wasn't so easy. I used to be a dedicated long-distance runner; with CFS, even five minutes of brisk walking could trigger pressure headaches and abnormal fatigue. How could this be? I walked to some extent throughout the day at work, certainly for more than a few minutes, but that didn't produce the immediate symptom flare-ups that I experienced when I did brisk walking. To me this was pathetic—I used to run like the wind.

Now I play volleyball for as long as one or two hours—without triggering symptom flare-ups, even though I may walk or run for brief spurts. On the face of it, there doesn't seem to be any underlying logic to why volleyball works for me but brisk walking does not. However, I now have some sense of why one activity causes problems, while another, perhaps more vigorous, activity does not.

I have discovered that for me, the healthy course is greater social connectedness and good relationships. Whenever I get too involved with solitary activities, whether it be running, walking, or sitting behind a computer, my symptoms increase. On the other hand, when I do limited physical activity in an enjoyable social context I experience no symptom flare-ups. And most importantly, when I take the time to improve my relationships, I feel healthier, both physically and emotionally.

The psyche controls, often unconsciously, the volume and intensity of illness. It's not a simple on/off switch; it's more like a valve that can adjust the gradation of illness, upward or downward depending on how you direct and balance your life. The primary goal of this book is to provide a road map of lifestyle changes that will give you greater control of that valve, thus leading to less impairment and reduced illness severity.

Studies of Poor Coping and Illness Worsening

What about the other side of the above list—the worsening illness side? How is coping related to illness worsening? Poor coping has frequently been associated with greater illness impairments in CFS. In the research literature, poor coping has generally been studied in terms of *catastrophizing* about the illness—viewing the illness as an all-encompassing plague-like event. For example, in the study conducted by Susan Buckelew (1996) described above, it was found that the FM patients who catastrophized the most were also the most disabled. Other studies have also shown that pessimistic attitudes and beliefs are correlated with increased disability and illness severity. A belief that your illness is uncontrollable results in a lessening of any effort to deal with symptoms. The abandonment of positive coping efforts also reduces opportunities for healthy contact with others and feelings of vitality.

Another form of poor coping is *denial of diagnosis*—devoting tremendous amounts of energy to pretending you're not ill. This typically involves persistent and forceful efforts not to think about your illness, and strenuous attempts to behave as much as possible like a healthy person. Although forced functioning based on fear and desperation may yield a surface reassurance that you aren't an invalid, a heavy toll is exacted: persistent fear leads to even greater exhaustion. Thus, although in the short term denial may keep you going, it's not a healthy solution.

■ Steve's Story: An Example of Catastrophizing

Steve suffered from chronic back pain and FM. His pain greatly worsened after an improperly done back surgery. Although Steve successfully sued for three million dollars, his ongoing pain prevented him from returning to work as a construction foreman.

His pain and limitations also prevented him from doing yard work—as well as almost any other vigorous activity. Moreover, his marriage was in trouble because he could no longer be a social or sexual partner to his wife. Understandably, he was very upset and depressed. Powerful pain-reducing narcotics caused him to be forgetful, easily angered, and almost zombie-like. Yet he preferred to take the medicine, rather than face the full force of the pain—and the likelihood of permanent disability. He was contemplating suicide.

However, a closer look at Steve's thinking revealed that he was actually aggravating his problems by viewing his life in all-or-nothing terms. Since he couldn't have his old job back—or something comparable—he rejected every other type of work. He looked all over the country for a physician to correct his back problem, but no surgeon would touch him because his back was so fragile after the previous surgery. Steve insisted that he had to be fixed and made whole, or else nothing mattered. With this kind of extreme, catastrophic thinking, is it any wonder that he was contemplating suicide?

In the course of two years of therapy, Steve realized that if he wanted to make his life work in any meaningful way, he would have to view his pain and limitations in a different way. And at last he began this process: rather than telling me every week that his pain was worse than the previous week, he instead began to focus on other things and do self-relaxation.

Just this one shift in his attention made a big difference. He looked more calm and composed in session. He complained much less and finally dropped his insistence that he be fixed before anything positive could happen. His relationship with his wife also improved. At this point he stopped therapy, so I don't know if he continued his improvements, but already the transformations in his attitude, demeanor, and his outlook were impressive.

Poor Coping and Despair

It's all too easy for people with CFS and FM to buy into the feelings of futility that arise out of chronic symptoms and view their lives as unbearable. I had this despairing attitude for many, many years: *I had to be made whole!* It's not the hope and desire to be well that gets you in trouble—it's the stubborn demand that you *must* be made well that leads to anger and depression and destructive coping. But you have a choice as to which beliefs you attach to your illness.

A physician colleague of mine was visited once a year by a patient with CFS, FM, and general disability. This patient only had one question when he came in: "Is there a cure yet?" With this question the patient revealed that he did little to help himself feel better physically or emotionally—he was entrenched in the belief that life was an intolerable burden as long as he had fatigue and pain. Of course, anyone with chronic fatigue and pain may feel like this sometimes; however, if your attitude becomes, "I am depending on a cure and nothing short of that will be satisfactory," then your life is on hold and you are wasting precious time in servitude to your pain.

In sum, we are inclined to get better with good coping and stress reduction, and inclined to get worse with poor coping and unrelieved stress. Fortunately, you can work on both simultaneously by increasing the good coping and reducing the bad coping. The skills of good coping can be learned by anyone and can be successfully applied in your daily schedule to reduce illness burdens. As these burdens lessen, illness improvements will begin.

Low-Level Stress: How It Worsens Illness

Stress is the ever-present companion of CFS and FM. You were probably stressed before you became ill. Then, at the beginning stages of illness, your stress most likely flared to overwhelming levels. These illnesses are particularly stress-sensitive; without recovery, stress becomes a persistent fact of life. The stress-symptom diaries that I ask my patients to keep for one or two weeks reveal a greatly increased sensitivity to the ordinary irritations and aggravations of everyday life.

To what extent does stress affect your overall condition? The greatest source of stress comes from the hassles of daily living; these hassles increase muscle tension, pain, and fatigue. However, you may not be fully aware of the impact of this daily, low-level stress on your well-being. You may mistakenly assume that it's your illness alone—and not daily hassles or stress—that keeps symptoms at high levels.

A diary study by Patrick Dailey et al. (1990) found that these routine hassles were actually more strongly related to FM symptoms than major life events. One reason for this may be because daily life hassles are with you continually while major life stress usually comes in dramatic bursts—e.g., divorce or bankruptcy or the death of a spouse. Of course, these major life events affect you as well, and I'm not attempting to minimize them; however, they're relatively rare compared to persistent daily stress.

You may be unaware of the low-level stress that you do experience. This is quite common in people with these illnesses—many have learned to ignore stress signals from their bodies, simply pushing on with their daily activities. Also, much of stress resides just below consciousness, so you may fail to recognize it or dismiss it because it's not obvious. However, even persistent, low-level stress can keep symptom levels higher than they would otherwise be.

Stress reduction techniques, another important tool in this improvement program, can reduce both stress flare-ups and the general stress that is always with you.

Why a Successful Improvement Program Takes Time

During the first eighteen years of my illness, I rejected the idea that stress or lifestyle could play any role in my illness. Because I could easily separate my emotional states (anxiety, depressed mood) from my CFS symptoms, I knew that these symptoms couldn't be explained by negative feelings alone. And the reality is that people with CFS and FM *are* ill apart from stress factors. However, the relationship of stress and lifestyle to these illnesses suggests that these factors play an important role in determining *how sick you are.*

I no longer reject the psychological literature that shows that coping and lifestyle are related to illness severity—and not just in CFS and FM, but in a variety of other medical conditions, including heart disease, cancer, lupus, and arthritis. However, this relationship may not be immediately obvious if you're trying this seven-step improvement program. Seeing improvement through lifestyle changes often requires several weeks to several months of planning and effort. Although not immediate, several weeks to several months is a very reasonable time frame for improvement, particularly given that many of us have already tried alternative treatments that involve commitments to vitamin therapies, diets, IV infusions, shots, and other exotica that can be roughly equal to part-time—or even full-time—work.

Those of you who have been ill for a long time, or who have tried any number of dubious treatment approaches, may find the techniques and principles of self-control described in the upcoming chapters particularly appealing. Why? Because the experience of setback after setback and disappointment after disappointment often leads to the important, bottom-line question: if nothing else seems to work, what can I change within myself?

What Is the Evidence for the Program?

This seven-step program is founded on proven cognitive behavioral therapy and stress reduction techniques. More than a dozen controlled scientific studies of cognitive behavioral treatment and graduated exercise programs for CFS and FM have consistently shown illness improvements, including symptom reductions and improved functioning. Overall, these behavioral treatments have worked for roughly two out of three individuals.

The techniques of cognitive behavioral therapy include gradually increasing or decreasing activity as tolerance develops, improving sleep, purging unrealistic fears of symptom flare-ups, and reducing the perfectionism that can drive one to the extremes of overwork and sacrifice. Additionally, published studies have shown that relaxation training has multiple benefits, particularly for those with FM, including significantly reduced illness impact, more restful sleep, and improved coping with symptoms.

PART II

The Seven Steps to Improvement

If you've invested any time in alternative or medical treatments, you've probably attempted to rate any improvements that might have resulted from those treatments. Often I hear people say that they may be somewhat better but they're not sure; sometimes, noticeable improvement will occur during the early stages of treatment only to be followed by a fallback to your usual illness state.

What Is Improvement?

If improvements are rated on a 100 percent scale with 0 being no change and 100 percent being completely well, a change of at least 20 percent indicates for most people a definite improvement. Changes of less than 20 percent are often difficult to judge, particularly given the normal fluctuations of these illnesses—perhaps you're slightly better, perhaps not.

On the other hand, if you see a rapid but short-lived improvement of greater than 20 percent from a particular treatment, this can probably be attributed to *placebo effect*. This doesn't mean you didn't actually experience that improvement, it means that the treatment isn't likely to be effective in the long term for any number of reasons. The placebo effect has to do with your hope and belief that a treatment will work.

Placebo Effects and Improvement

The placebo effect is a well-documented phenomenon in medical treatment studies; it has occurred in medication studies ranging from high blood pressure to hair loss. For example, people with hypertension will show some health benefit from taking an inactive pill if they believe they are getting an effective treatment for their blood pressure. Even studies of the hair loss remedy minoxidil showed that some men grew hair simply after rubbing an inactive placebo lotion into their bald spots. This demonstrates how powerful belief and expectation can be in affecting bodily processes. Placebo effects are evident in treatment studies of CFS and FM as well.

The placebo response does not indicate weakness of character or suggestibility or any other negative trait. It is simply a fact of the human condition—everyone is subject to placebo influences on their condition. If I could simply believe I was getting better, without effective treatment, and that could in and of itself make me well, I wouldn't have a problem with that. Of course, it's not so simple.

Improvement with the Seven-Step Program

If you follow the lifestyle and stress reduction recommendations in this book for at least six months—following the recommendations to the letter—you will experience a noticeable improvement in your condition. And by noticeable improvement I mean an improvement of at least 20 percent and perhaps much greater. I have seen improvements 50 percent or greater—and in some cases, even near recovery.

If you do less than the full program but show no improvement, you really can't accurately judge if the full program would have worked for you. You may need to do *all* seven steps to get improvements (although you may find over time that certain steps are much more important for you to maintain). Simply trying a single technique on its own for a week and then deciding it doesn't have much effect will shortchange you of the program's potential benefits.

Thus, to ensure the greatest likelihood of improvement, I strongly urge you to do all seven steps. The people with these illnesses who have been able to improve most have all made major changes to their personal belief systems, behaviors, and their ability to manage stress in their daily lives. The seven steps will help you, too, to make these types of changes.

Devoting your personal efforts to illness improvement also means that you depend less on the (not so almighty) medical and alternative treatments. The more you depend on external treatments, the less patience you will have to examine and reevaluate your life. I'm not saying that external treatments should be completely abandoned, but they should be viewed for what they are: a way to manage symptoms more or less temporarily, not a cure. After all, if your physical treatments were that beneficial I doubt that you'd be reading this book!

I'm not preaching a complete recovery protocol here, only a path to improvement and possibly near recovery for some (I put myself in this category). A complete, sustained recovery (or cure) probably requires medical therapies as yet undiscovered.

A Balanced Life: The Key Factor in Improvement

The severity of your illness is related to how far out of balance your lifestyle is. The more focused you are on stressful activities to the exclusion of stress-reducing activities, the more severe your illness is likely to be. On the other hand, the more effort you make to do stress-reducing and mood-uplifting activities, the less intrusive and less severe your illness will become. The bottom line is achieving balance in your life, no matter how sick or disabled you may be.

For the most active, this means reducing overwork and increasing the amount of enjoyable leisure time. For the least active, this means increasing activity levels and reducing stress. And for those in between these two extremes, it means rearranging your lifestyle so that stress is reduced and pleasure is increased.

CHAPTER 7

Step One: Using Active, Extended Relaxation Strategies

Like many people with CFS and FM, you've probably learned to respect your body—you may watch what you eat or take pains to reduce your exposure to allergens and toxic chemicals; but you probably don't give the stress in your life the same level of attention or care. However, you can achieve benefits that equal—and often exceed—those that come from healthy diets and clean environments simply by reducing the negative effects of stress on your body.

Unhealthy stress is often the result of overextended lifestyles that involve overwork and over-responsibility—a kind of work hard/play hard mentality that allows little time for leisure, contemplation, and pleasant relaxing experiences. For people with CFS and FM, deep relaxation can seem like an unnatural state of being—it may conjure up ideas about laziness, badness, and sloth.

Of course you'd prefer your lifestyle to be active and bustling. As one person with CFS put it, there's nothing more rewarding than the "euphoria of accomplishment." But there's a big price to be paid for nonstop activity: putting out all that energy without taking time for yourself means you stay exhausted.

Relaxation-Based Improvement

The ability to relax is an important coping skill. Regular relaxation exercises can give you a sense of control over your illness—and as discussed in chapter 6, studies on coping in CFS and FM have found that a sense of control over symptoms consistently predicts better functioning, regardless of limitations or disabilities.

Do you take the time to relax now that you are ill? You may think you do—I thought I did—but you're probably carrying around a lot more tension and stress than you realize. Will a little relaxation help? Probably. Will massive amounts help even more? Definitely.

■ Jim's Story: Relaxation Effects in a Person with CFS

Jim, a forty-three-year-old engineer, was diagnosed with CFS a year before he contacted me. Previously, he had worked sixty-hour weeks and done vigorous aerobic exercise regularly but had devoted little time to either his relationship with his wife and child or to leisurely pursuits. His illness was apparently triggered by an adverse reaction to several abrupt changes in his asthma medication. After Jim began to experience near-constant flu-like symptoms and profound physical fatigue, he had to quit all work except for five hours a week of home-based consultation.

Initially, Jim was very nervous about his limitations and the future of his marriage; he wondered if his independent-minded wife could accept a new role as a caregiver to him. Given his pervasive feelings of foreboding, I focused on relaxation techniques to reduce his stress. Because Jim had done relaxation exercises sporadically for ten years, I suggested that he now practice them regularly, twice a day, for thirty minutes each time. He did, and experienced some level of calm during the relaxation exercise itself but found that the feeling quickly faded afterward. I asked him to double his relaxation time and see what happened. With the increased time, the relaxation experience deepened and began to carry over into his nonmeditation hours, and Jim's anxieties about being ill lessened as well.

He then further increased the relaxation sessions, to two hours a day. As a result, he experienced an even more enduring calm—and much less fear about his future. At the same time, he was also changing his long-standing beliefs about work: work was no longer an irrevocable part of his identity, no longer his road to salvation. Instead, he began to think of work as something important that he used to do but didn't *have* to do again. This was a profound change in Jim's view of his life.

His focus now became improving his health as much as possible through his own personal efforts. His relationship with his wife also improved; although previously he'd viewed her as a less than ideal partner, he now recognized the practical day-to-day support she provided. And he was much more openly appreciative of her efforts as a result.

Would these changes have occurred without the extended relaxation sessions? I can't answer that question with certainty, but the positive changes all happened when Jim increased his daily relaxation time. And they occurred quickly. This wasn't a gradual change in Jim's thinking or a slow change that might happen to anyone who is ill for a long time. This was an uplifting transformation. My belief is that relaxation was a key factor in Jim's ability to positively transform his attitudes about work and marriage.

The Positive Effects of Relaxation

Relaxation is to CFS and FM what aspirin is to headaches; relaxation can reduce symptoms and dissolve tension. Although sometimes these effects may only last for a few minutes (perhaps just long enough to get through a particularly stressful situation), other times these effects can last for hours. Tranquilizing medication may be helpful for some individuals, but no medication can substitute for good stress management.

I've practiced meditation techniques for over twenty years and at this point I feel almost permanently relaxed (although I do still get tense at times). I remember how much more emotional I used to be before starting my two decades of self-relaxation: I used to be tense and easy to anger—although I never expressed it. Much of the time I just simmered with anger—anger at injustice, anger at unfairness, anger at any bad thing that happened to me. My immediate reaction to any adversity was anger.

Meditation has uprooted most of my anger: I may still think angry thoughts, but I never feel the all-consuming rage that I used to. You, too, can achieve this kind of easing of your negative emotions; it's not that you'll be less aware of your negative emotions, it's just that you'll be less affected by them.

A number of studies on relaxation techniques have demonstrated the benefits of regular relaxation practice, including:

- Stress reduction

- Reduction in muscular tension

- Diminished anxiety and worry

- Increased sense of well-being

- Lessened pain

What may be especially relevant to CFS and FM is that regular relaxation practice has been shown to improve some aspects of immune function (see chapter 2 about immune function aberrations as a possible causal factor in both illnesses).

How Much Relaxation Is Needed?

For much of my two decades of relaxation practice, I meditated twice a day, for twenty minutes at a time. Before I became ill, this daily meditation practice gave rise to very pleasurable feelings of calm that lasted through much of the day. After I became ill, however, the meditation did not work so well: relaxation-induced good feelings were reduced and didn't last as long. As a result, I came to view my daily meditation practice as a good coping skill to reduce stress and negative feelings in general, but nothing more—I certainly didn't view it as an illness reduction technique.

Extended Relaxation Studies in FM

Then, in March 2001, I read a press release (*Psychosomatic Medicine*, 2001) about an interesting relaxation study in people with FM. Two psychologists, Sandra Sephton and Paul Salman, conducted a well-designed study and presented their findings at the annual meeting of the American Psychosomatic Society. Ninety women were involved in the trial. Half were assigned to a four-month group meditation and stress reduction program while the other half were put on a wait list and didn't receive any training. Those in the group program were helped to develop a routine involving daily meditation that lasted forty-five minutes to an hour a day, six days a week.

Sephton and Salman found that the patients who had meditated regularly were significantly less depressed, less sleep-deprived, and less affected by their illness than those who hadn't meditated. Also, the patients who meditated showed healthy changes in their levels of the stress hormone cortisol. Sephton and Salman concluded that meditation can help FM patients both by reducing stress and changing the way the body reacts to stressful situations, and suggested that people with FM could benefit—twenty-four hours a day—from a single hour of meditation, in much the same way that thirty to forty-five minutes of aerobic exercise a day benefits the heart, even at rest.

"We looked at how your body responds to stress in general when you're not meditating," noted Sephton, "and the research shows that meditation sort of dampens down your physiological response to stress even when you're not meditating, so you benefit the next time you're in traffic: instead of getting high blood pressure you deal with it better physiologically."

These researchers did caution, however, that meditation appears to help only those who are committed to regular practice of stress reduction techniques. "One hour a day meditation requires a lot of effort on the part of the patient," noted Salman. "And it is only the people who use these techniques regularly who show this decrease in their stress response."

Another study done more than a decade ago with FM patients also suggests that relaxation is related to illness improvement (Kaplan,

Goldenberg, and Galvin-Nadeau 1993). After a ten-week group meditation-based stress reduction program, 51 percent of the seventy-seven patients showed moderate to marked improvement in terms of well-being, sleep, pain, and fatigue. Perhaps you are surprised and skeptical—how can something as simple as relaxation techniques produce such great improvements? Well, the reasons may have to do with the study design itself: patients met every week in a group to discuss what they did. This built into the study both week-to-week accountability and support from the group for the daily practice of meditation. Normally you won't receive such high levels of support to take time for yourself.

To achieve the good results of these FM meditation studies, it may require several weeks of regular daily relaxation practice, not just an occasional deep breath when you feel stressed or symptomatic. If you take that time it also indicates that you have put positive leisure time in your life, something that many people with CFS and FM do only rarely. To be successful, you need to convince yourself that these techniques are not a waste of time. Relaxation will ultimately become something you *want* to do because of the benefits it provides. If you think of it only as something you should do, it will lose much of its power to help you.

Increasing Your Relaxation Time

Intrigued by the findings of these studies, I increased my two daily relaxation periods from twenty minutes to thirty minutes each. I then had to overcome a certain feeling of annoyance about devoting even more time to relaxation, but once I did, benefits came quickly. Within the first two days, I experienced feelings of greater tolerance, greater well-being, and less irritability throughout the day. I was also more tolerant of my symptom flare-ups and less concerned about any kind of timetable for improving. I focused, instead, on how I could function my best without increasing my symptoms.

My new level of calm also helped me to realize how tense I'd become in certain situations. For example, I now noticed that the pressure I put on myself to play well in my weekly volleyball games actually interfered with my playing. I used to think that a certain competitive pressure was necessary to keep me motivated. However, after two weeks on this new relaxation schedule, this pressure was reduced almost to nothing; absent was the urgency to play every shot well, absent was the worry that I might shank the ball. When I played my shots, I played them much more calmly—and as a result, I could use the split seconds between shots to plan how to hit the ball. I played better and enjoyed myself more.

An important point about the volleyball is that I hadn't even realized how my own stress was interfering with my enjoyment. I think very few people with CFS and FM realize how much low-level stress and tension interferes with their good feelings. Or, as another way of saying it, that their stress prevents good feelings from being as strong as they could be.

Did the increased amounts of relaxation reduce my illness severity in general? It's difficult to give a definitive answer because relaxation, good feelings, and illness severity are all related to some degree. As in the FM relaxation studies, the illness and its effects (poor sleep, irritability) now had much less impact on me. If the illness affects you much less, is that the same as less illness? This is a conundrum with no easy answer. But does it really matter? If you significantly shrink the impact of the illness on your life, isn't that a valuable improvement in and of itself? Of course, if you insist on a cure, on an all-or-none outcome, then no improvement, short of recovery, is ever enough. But that attitude only leads to endless frustration and despair. Which track do you want to be on? You decide.

Relaxation Techniques

Many relaxation techniques have been developed to target physical, mental, emotional, and spiritual aspects of the stress reduction process. Which technique(s) you decide to use is largely a matter of personal preference, ease of use, and effectiveness.

Breathing Focus

I would start with a simple and very effective technique. First, sit in a comfortable chair or lie down. Now, say silently to yourself a long "reee" as you inhale—and then a slow "laaax" as you exhale. Your breathing should be natural. Avoid taking more than one or two deep breaths or breathing out of your mouth; breathing normally through your nose is easiest. To start, do the relaxation before meals, ten minutes in the morning and ten minutes in the late afternoon. (Choose a time when you can expect a minimum of interruptions from family or others and minimize your distractions—e.g., turn off the phone/turn on the answering machine.)

Progressive Muscular Relaxation

Particularly for people with FM who experience significant pain, I recommend an additional relaxation technique called *progressive muscular relaxation* (this can be alternated with the breathing focus technique described above). Many people with FM are unaware of how much they are tensing their muscles. This series of tension-relaxation exercises makes them aware of both their level of tension and the relaxation that they can feel.

The instructions for the following progressive muscular relaxation exercise have been written out fully so that you—or a friend—can read them into a recording device first, thus allowing you to then listen and do the exercises without any interruptions. Alternatively, I have prepared a 45-minute relaxation tape (or CD) that you can order (see the resources section at the end of the book for ordering information). This tape contains the breathing focus technique and a full set of progressive muscular relaxation exercises, as well as some guided imagery suggestions (this technique will be discussed later in the chapter). Each progressive relaxation exercise should be done twice before going onto the next exercise.

Get comfortable in a soft chair. Legs and arms should be uncrossed.

Focus on your right hand.

Make a fist. Keep the rest of your body relaxed. Let the tension grow. (8 seconds)

Now let it go. The muscles go limp; there is nothing you have to do. Let the tension begin to flow away.

Sink into relaxation. (15 seconds)

Focus on your left hand.

Make a tight fist with your left hand, keeping the rest of your body relaxed. Let the tension build. (8 seconds)

Now let it go. Let the tension flow out. Let the feelings of tension dissolve. Become limp and loose. Relax. (15 seconds)

Focus on your right arm.

Squeeze your lower and your upper arm together; try to touch your wrist to your shoulder. (8 seconds)

Squeeze tighter and tighter. Notice the feelings of tension.

Let go. The tension melts away. The muscles become more deeply relaxed. (15 seconds)

Now focus on your left arm.

Squeeze your lower and upper arm together. Tighten it. Tighten the muscles, let the tension build. (8 seconds)

And let go. As the tension flows away, your muscles begin to smooth over, you begin to unwind. Sink deeper and deeper into relaxation. (15 seconds)

Focus on the muscles in the back of your neck.

Slowly tilt your head back and gently squeeze your neck muscles. Let the tension grow, into a full, complete squeeze. (8 seconds)

Gently let go. Let your muscles go completely limp. Tension dissolves, flows away. (15 seconds)

Focus on your shoulders.

Raise your shoulders into a high shrug. Feel tension across the shoulders and the back of the neck. Feel that tension. Experience it. (8 seconds)

Release. Let the shoulders return to a resting, comfortable position. As the tension flows away, experience the sensations of relaxation, more and more. (15 seconds)

Focus on your jaw.

Press your molars together—not too hard—and clench the muscles of your jaw together. Feel the tension. (8 seconds)

Release. Let the jaw slacken. Feel the jaw become loose and limp. (15 seconds)

Focus on your eyes.

Open your eyes very wide. Raise your eyebrows and wrinkle up your forehead. Hold that tension, hold it. (8 seconds)

And release. Let the eye muscles return to a resting, comfortable position. Let the forehead become smooth. The eyes soften, feelings of tension fade away. (15 seconds)

Now, close your eyes tightly, tightly. Feel the tension. Hold onto it, hold it. (8 seconds)

And release. Feel the tension disappear, let the eyes return to a comfortable position, relaxation flowing in. Feel the release of tension. More and more, feel that release of tension. (15 seconds)

Focus on your shoulders.

Push your shoulders back, moving your shoulder blades closer together. Squeeze your shoulder blades even closer together. Feel the tension in your back, hold onto it. (8 seconds)

And release. Let the tension go, let the back muscles release. Feel that release of tension. More and more, feel that release of tension. (15 seconds)

Focus on your right leg.

Tense the muscles of your right leg. Tense them up. Feel that tension. If you're sitting, push your right foot into the floor. Experience the tension. Let it grow. (8 seconds)

Let it go. Let the right leg become looser and looser; feel these loosening sensations as you sink deeper and deeper into relaxation. (15 seconds)

Now focus on your left leg.

Tense the muscles of your left leg. Tense them up. Feel that tension. If you're sitting, push your left foot into the floor. Experience the tension. Let it grow. (8 seconds)

Let it go. Let the left leg become looser and looser; feel these loosening sensations as you sink deeper and deeper into relaxation. (15 seconds)

Now, slowly, gradually, bring yourself to wakefulness. Gradually allow yourself to return to a relaxed wakefulness. Feel relaxed and refreshed as you slowly become more alert.

Pause 15–30 seconds before standing up.

Imagery

Another relaxation technique is guided imagery, such as focusing on beach, mountain, or country scenes. (Similar to the previous progressive muscular relaxation technique, you may find it easiest to read the following beach imagery exercise into a recording device first, and then allow yourself to listen to it without interruption.)

Imagine yourself at the beach. The sand feels warm and soft against your skin as you sit watching the ocean. You observe the azure blue water, you watch the waves as they move rhythmically to the shore, the water becoming a light transparent green as it flows to the shore-line. You see the whitecaps of the waves as the waves roll onto the shore; yes, waves gently reaching the shore, sparkling water spilling on the sand. You feel a salty, refreshing spray in the air, a refreshing, misty spray all over your body, wonderfully invigorating and uplifting; revitalizing and relaxing.

Allow yourself the next few moments to imagine the pleasant flow of the waves onto the shore as they rise and fall, rise and fall. Imagine the waves. (Pause for about 5 seconds.)

All right. Very good. Now, you decide to take an easy stroll along the beach as you watch the surf. Observe the curving shoreline off in the distance, the curving shoreline as it merges with the horizon. As you walk onward, onward, you feel the sand crunching beneath your feet; such a pleasant sensation; warm, crunchy sand. It complements the warmth of the sun overhead. Feel the gentle warmth of the sun on your back, that gentle warmth flowing down your back and throughout your body; the comfortable, gentle warmth from the sun fills you with pleasant sensations. With your senses so very aware, you notice the sand dunes rising along the beach, sand dunes with isolated clumps of tall grass on their slopes. Observe the tall grass gently sway in the breeze. The breezes create tranquil feelings.

As you walk onward, you hear the sound of seagulls in the distance. A flock of white seagulls approaches, flying easily, gliding in the wind, squawking as they pass overhead. Now they're flying off into the distance, leaving you with a feeling of serenity. A gentle ocean breeze slips softly across your back. The gentle breeze coaxes you further along, heightens your senses.

As you look across the waves, you see a sleek white sailboat moving through the water. The boat moves so gracefully, the sails filled with gently sweeping winds. Enjoy the silent steadiness of the boat as it slips along with the wind.

Now, as you gaze toward the horizon, you see the sun setting. Yes, a sunset, with a full display of vivid colors: bright yellows, deep reds, and burnt oranges, all against light gray clouds and pale blue sky. As the sun descends, it shines a long wedge of yellow light across the water. Slowly the sun sinks down. A breathtaking serenity begins to pervade the atmosphere, an emerging serenity so deep that it fully absorbs your senses.

You begin to conclude now. Finish the experience with acceptance and peace, acceptance and peace. Allow yourself all the time in the world, all the time you need, to bring yourself back to wakefulness. Let your eyes open slowly, feeling relaxed and refreshed.

Other Forms of Relaxation

Although breathing focus and guided imagery are probably the simplest forms of self-relaxation, other forms of more active relaxation can also produce very good results. It's important to find a relaxation exercise that's compatible with your needs and preferences. If you have the energy, relaxation feelings can be increased by combining light stretching or light yoga exercises prior to the breathing-based or imagery-based relaxation. Physical and mental relaxation complement each other: the stretching results in a sense of muscular loosening and flexibility while the mental relaxation creates a sense of calm and tranquility. Together, they produce a deep, overall calming effect.

Other forms of relaxation include muscular training, autogenic training, prayer, long peaceful baths, and listening to soothing music. To achieve improvement-level benefits, the same guidelines apply: you must practice the technique an hour a day and it must produce a relaxation experience, called an *R-state*. (R-states are explained at greater length in the next section.)

If the relaxation techniques in this chapter don't work for you even after you've practiced them diligently, try an alternative technique. If you continue to experience difficulties, consider taking a more formal class.

R-States, Relaxation, and Improvement

Relaxation states—R-states—are the physical and mental experiences that occur during relaxation exercises that make them so effective and rewarding. R-states aren't simply on/off feelings that are either present or absent; R-states can be present in varying degrees, depending on the other things you may be doing. Relaxation that is matched to the task at hand will actually increase productivity. For example, if you're working on your computer you probably wouldn't want to feel profound sleepiness—that would interfere with your work. On the other hand, if your attention to your task is accompanied by a general sense of ease and comfort, you're that much less likely to be distracted by irrelevant worries, frustrations, and background noise.

The R-state concept was conceived by psychologist Jonathan Smith (1990), a specialist in relaxation techniques. Let's take a look at the world of R-states—try to identify which of the sensations listed below you experience during your relaxation exercises. (As you identify these sensations, you can also contrast them with the routine daily stressors that dampen your pleasant feelings; as you become more and more aware of the contrast between R-states and stressful feelings, you can bring about the R-states more easily and make them part of your daily life. The more you experience R-states, the better you will feel—and the less impact your illness will have on your life.)

Examples of R-States

R-states may include:

- Lightness or heaviness

- Warmth or coolness

- Pleasant tingling or numbness

- Physical relaxation

- Mental relaxation

- Mental quiet

- Sleepiness

- Strength and awareness

- Joy

- Love and thankfulness

- Prayerfulness

These R-states are pleasant feelings that individuals with CFS and FM rarely experience because they are so seldom relaxed. Many people with these illnesses only experience R-states fleetingly, perhaps as occasional bouts of sleepiness during the day, or physical relaxation after some physical activity—e.g., sex or yard work. Other R-states, such as mental quiet and mental relaxation, are often completely unfamiliar to people with CFS and FM, particularly those who have highly active minds and trouble turning them off. These R-states are a unique blend of calm and quiet—a kind of peaceful silence sometimes experienced without any thoughts.

When you first start to feel relaxation effects, you'll probably experience one or more of the first four R-states on the list. Once your tensions have been calmed through regular practice of relaxation techniques, you may then experience the higher levels of R-states. You may feel such R-states as joy, love, and thankfulness—and, in special deep moments, prayerful reverence.

The Importance of R-States

R-states are necessary for relaxation to work. No matter how much you practice relaxation, if your relaxation techniques don't evoke at least some R-states, you're wasting your time. Similarly, no matter how many years you spend in yoga or meditation classes, if you're not experiencing at least some R-states, you're wasting your money. If you don't experience R-states, you're unlikely to get relaxation's health benefits.

The Profound Benefits of Extended Relaxation and Meditation

Those who incorporate an hour—or more—of deep relaxation into their day will often experience benefits far beyond the relaxation session itself. The peace and serenity that develops within the session can become the foundation for a more relaxed attitude toward life and accomplishment in general. In my experience, when individuals who are disabled with CFS and FM devote this level of time to active relaxation, they often begin to experience their lives in a more positive and appreciative way—whether in terms of improved relationships, greater self-acceptance, or a greater appreciation of the small things that can still be accomplished.

Another benefit of relaxation is that it teaches you to become more aware of your body's reactions to stress and illness. This awareness in and of itself helps address and counteract the negative tendency that many people with these illnesses have to either ignore physical symptoms or dwell anxiously on them.

Relaxation helps to both identify and release the stress you experience. Each relaxation session is a process of cleansing and renewal. When it works really well relaxation allows you to rethink unhealthy habits and reactions. And the health benefits of relaxation itself are well established scientifically. You need only to prove them to yourself through the direct experience.

■ Elizabeth's Story: One Woman's Benefits from Relaxation

Elizabeth, a thirty-five-year-old divorced woman with FM, experienced widespread body pain, aching, and stiffness. Any kind of lifting caused pain flare-ups. As a result, she no longer had the energy to do her highly physical work as a maintenance supervisor and had to stop work. In a stress reduction group for people with FM, she was given home relaxation exercises. After several weeks of practicing the exercises, her worries about the future lessened—and she replaced her worries with plans to live a simpler life. This included good relationships, low-level physical activities, and more leisure time for herself. At her last group session, she described how, while watching a good movie, she had felt completely pain-free for roughly two hours—the first time that had happened since she became ill.

Setting Up a Relaxation Schedule

I suggest that you start with ten to twenty minutes of relaxation, twice a day, for the first two weeks and then, in the third week of your relaxation program, increase that to thirty minutes twice a day. Although even twenty minutes a day of active relaxation is better than none, I consider an hour a day the bare minimum necessary to put your illness on the improvement track. If you have the time, I strongly recommend that you increase your daily relaxation time to an hour in the morning and an hour in the afternoon or evening (or divide it into four half-hour blocks).

If you find yourself reacting with horror to the idea of so much relaxation, design your relaxation schedule so that it fits into your day rather than interferes with it. For instance, if you have more energy in the morning and want to use it for activities other than relaxation, put your relaxation practice time in during the afternoon and evening. Alternatively, if you have trouble sleeping, it's probably better to bunch up your relaxation time in the evening (see chapter 8). Also, you don't have to divide your relaxation into two thirty-minute blocks—you can spread mini-relaxation periods throughout your day instead. Say, a minute here, two minutes there. It will still add up and provide a more continuous feeling of calm. I know many people—including myself—who do this and still get all the benefits of two long relaxation sessions.

You may also wish to purchase relaxation audio recordings to create some variety in your relaxation experience. Mine can only be ordered directly from me (see the resources section at the end of the book), but many other relaxation tapes and CDs are also now available in bookstores, pharmacies, and other retail outlets.

The beneficial effects of relaxation will pay you back in terms of improved quality of life. Specifically, you'll be able to accomplish tasks with less stress, less pain, and even somewhat less fatigue. You'll also then conserve more energy because you're doing things in a more relaxed manner.

One thirty-eight-year-old woman with FM described how relaxation helped her thus:

> *I learned a relaxation technique in a special class, which was okay, but practicing it at home was a pain at first. There are so many other things I have to do! But by doing the relaxation I began to realize how stressed I was just doing all my housework and taking care of the kids when they got home. The relaxation helped me get off the daily treadmill. It lessened some of the exhaustion I feel. I also feel less irritable and snappy with the kids, which has been a big problem since I got sick.*

If, despite all of my arguments, you are not convinced to do daily relaxation, please go on to the next chapter. Although relaxation is very important, you can still benefit—and improve—using the remaining steps. But remember: the more fully you do each step, the greater your chances for improvement.

CHAPTER 8

Step Two: Sleeping Better, Relaxing More

Sleep disturbance is common in CFS and FM. Poor sleep patterns can take any number of forms, from difficulty in falling asleep (or staying asleep) to early morning awakenings to restless, agitated sleep.

Improving sleep involves making your environment as conducive to good sleep as possible. Although many of the suggestions I give will seem like common sense, the idea is to put together a sleep *program* for yourself that involves changing your sleep habits overall. Doing one or two things here and there will probably not improve your sleep. The program requires some level of thought, planning, and effort; however, often even after just a brief trial of a few days your sleep will begin to improve.

Study of Sleep Improvement in People with Chronic Pain

Although no study has focused specifically on improving sleep in people with CFS and FM, a recent treatment study (Currie, Wilson, and Curran 2002) focused on sleep problems in sixty people with chronic pain. The study's therapy consisted of seven weeks of group sessions aimed at promoting good sleep habits, teaching relaxation skills, and changing negative thoughts about sleep. By the end of the study, treated participants were significantly more improved than control participants in several ways: they fell asleep more quickly, they were awake less during the night, and their overall quality of sleep was better. Those who improved also demonstrated less restlessness during sleep, as measured by objective recording devices. These good results were maintained at a three-month follow-up.

You may ask, "Why should I put any effort into sleeping better? I slept fine without any effort before I became ill. Maybe sleep medications are better. At least they would be quick and easy." If sleep medications normalize your sleep, then maybe you don't need to do anything more. But for many, these drugs either don't work or have bad side effects. Or they may lose their effectiveness over time. Also, we don't currently know the long-term effects of taking sleep medications regularly. The bottom line is that only you can improve your sleep patterns on a consistent basis. Yes, it takes effort. But if you follow the suggestions in this chapter, your sleep will almost certainly improve, perhaps to a large degree. And as a result, you'll feel more rested and alert during the day—and you won't have the added burden of poor sleep to worsen your illness.

Start with Good Sleep Hygiene

The following sleep hygiene suggestions are useful in improving your sleep-wake patterns so that day and night are well-differentiated:

Stick to a Schedule

It's important to go to sleep and wake up at regular times. Your internal sleep-wake clock regulates the important hormonal patterns of melatonin, cortisol, and serotonin. When your sleep-wake clock is properly set, these hormones help you stay alert and awake during the day—and maintain good sleep at night. However, your illness has probably disrupted these hormonal patterns. Keeping regular hours for going to sleep and waking up in the morning will start the process of resetting the sleep-wake clock and help you to get better sleep. A regular bedtime hour also makes it easier to set up a time for wind-down activities.

Limit Your Bed Activities

It's important to make distinctions between day behavior (waking activities) and night behavior (lying down and sleeping). Use your bed for sleep and sexual activities only. For example, if you eat and watch TV in bed, these waking activities can become associated with lying in bed and interfere with healthy sleep patterns.

Stop Daytime Napping

Limit or eliminate daytime napping altogether. The more you nap in the daytime, the more difficult it becomes for your body to differentiate between day and night behavioral patterns. As much as you can, cut down on any napping during the day.

Eliminating naps may be very difficult—if not impossible—for those people whose energy level hovers around zero. Still, as an alternative to napping, try daytime resting with active relaxation, perhaps in a comfortable chair or recliner.

Change Your Clothes

If you're at home for much or most of the day, wear daytime clothes in your waking hours and pajamas for sleep. This, too, will help your body differentiate between day behavioral patterns and night behavioral patterns.

Easing the Active Mind with Wind-Down Activities

Many people with CFS and FM complain that—despite profound physical fatigue—they cannot shut their minds off at night. It's a problem often described as "tired and wired." (This complaint is also common among chronically poor sleepers and insomniacs.) A one-hour wind-down routine can dampen mental overactivity and help you drift off into sleep. Wind-down activities can be undertaken in whatever form you prefer, whether it be reading, listening to music, or practicing relaxation techniques. (Although watching TV may be mentally numbing, it's not necessarily relaxing, and I would recommend against it as a wind-down technique.) Physically and mentally active things should be avoided during the wind-down period, from housecleaning to phone calls to intense discussions. And, of course, caffeine should also be avoided as much as possible—particularly during the evening.

The goal of your bedtime wind-down routine is to fully relax and distance yourself from stressful or exciting thoughts. These thoughts might include worries or plans for the next day—or even interesting but overly stimulating thoughts. Both categories of thoughts will increase mental arousal and keep you awake.

Tired vs. Sleepy

When you use wind-down activities to relax at night, you'll also induce sleepiness. Sleepiness is different from tiredness and fatigue. Although you may be tired much of the time, you may feel sleepy only occasionally—perhaps during the day when you don't want to sleep. Feelings of sleepiness, especially if induced by relaxation, will lead to more restful sleep. Tiredness alone will not have this effect.

Use Extended Relaxation

I strongly recommend practicing an extended relaxation technique before bed. This means a good thirty minutes—or more—of extended relaxation, whether by the breathing focus technique, progressive muscular relaxation, guided imagery, or some other technique (see chapter 7).

If these techniques fail to produce substantial relaxation, you may want to try a commercially available relaxation tape or a sound machine (See Resource section at the end of this book for my relaxation tape.). Relaxation tapes usually describe calming scenarios, such as the beach, mountains, or countryside; sound machines now have settings for a number of relaxing situations. As the relaxation procedure continues, you'll feel less and less tense and sleepiness will drift over you. If you're still awake when the tape ends, continue to say the "relax" phrase to yourself until you doze off to sleep. Or simply play the tape again. Some people need the ongoing and powerful distraction of a tape to get away from their thoughts and ease into sleep.

People with CFS and FM who have trouble falling asleep—or staying asleep—often find that a ten- to fifteen-minute relaxation exercise doesn't help them. However, when they double their relaxation time, many then find that the relaxation exercises do actually help them fall asleep more easily and feel more rested the next day. (You can do a nighttime relaxation session as one of your two daily relaxation sessions. The amount of total daily relaxation—provided it's an hour or more—will still produce the benefits described in chapter 7.)

When you fall asleep feeling relaxed mentally and physically, you sleep more restfully—and sleep longer into the night without waking up. This is particularly important for people with CFS and FM, because people with these illnesses are chronically tense and tension is incompatible with restful sleep. I recommend practicing wind-down relaxation, *even if you fall asleep quickly*—it will program both a more restful sleep and fewer nighttime awakenings.

■ Fran's Story: An Example of Improved Sleep with Relaxation

Fran, a fifty-seven-year-old woman with FM, used a taped relaxation procedure to wind down at night. As a result, she had some nights of good sleep; however, on other nights she hardly slept at all. She decided to try a low dose of an antidepressant drug (amitriptyline) and an herbal supplement for sleep; they didn't help. In fact, one time, the combination of these two substances actually caused her to collapse to her knees—frightening her so much that she stopped both medications.

I advised her to use the progressive muscular relaxation exercise—an exercise that's particularly effective in reducing persistent but unrecognized muscle tension—immediately followed by the relaxation tape. In one week, this new relaxation procedure began to allow her to sleep more consistently. In particular, she noticed the difference between the tension and relaxation phases of the new relaxation technique and experienced relaxed feelings that were much deeper than before—feelings that helped her drift into sleepiness much more easily.

Handling Wake-Ups

Now, despite the use of extended relaxation before bed, you may still wake up during the night and have difficulty falling back asleep. If you do wake up during the night, use your preferred relaxation technique to ease yourself back into a sleepy state. (If you listen to an audiotape, use headphones if the sound bothers your spouse.) These simple relaxation techniques will allow you to feel better in the morning and through the next day, even if your sleep is not substantially better. Relaxation itself gives you greater feelings of well-being—a feeling particularly important to have when you're burdened by poor sleep.

If you're having trouble sleeping, I ask that you lie in bed awake for no longer than thirty minutes. This applies both to when you first go to sleep and when you wake up in the middle of the night. Why? Because in order to reestablish the association between your bed and sleeping, you need to use your bed for sleeping only (with the exception of sexual activity). If, when you get into bed at night for sleep, you aren't asleep after thirty minutes, you're probably not sleepy yet, only tired or exhausted.

When you get up after thirty minutes of nonsleep, do a quiet activity—such as reading or relaxing—in another room until you feel at least the beginnings of sleepiness. (A relaxation technique while sitting in a comfortable chair may help coax you into a sleepy state.) Then get back into bed. Once again, if you're not asleep in about thirty minutes, get out of bed and do a quiet activity. If your sleep is very disturbed, you may find this routine highly frustrating, but a number of studies show that this is one of the most effective sleep induction techniques there is. You should start seeing results in two to five days.

■ Kathy's Story: Using the Get-Up Technique

Kathy, who had CFS and FM for five years, often grew frustrated by the poor quality of her sleep. Typically, she would go to sleep at 11:00 P.M., only to wake up at 5:00 A.M. unable to return to sleep. She would then toss and turn for several hours, feeling very frustrated. After several months of this poor sleep pattern, she discovered that frustration was not the only way to react to poor sleep. She decided to get up at 5:00 A.M., use a half hour of quiet time to play solitaire, and then do some light housecleaning before the rest of the family woke up. Also, she began taking a two-hour nap in the afternoon, which she found restful and refreshing. (I know: good sleep hygiene discourages naps. However, you do also have to individualize your self-help—sometimes this involves utilizing certain guidelines and ignoring others.)

As a result of these changes, Kathy realized that her early morning frustration had been worsening her mood and her CFS symptoms. Her new schedule eliminated her early morning frustration—and caused her to think much less about her fatigue and poor sleep overall. As a result, she was less preoccupied with her fatigue and malaise and could focus instead on being productive and feeling well—yet another example of the mind-body connection in CFS and its powerful influence on your mood and your symptoms.

Some Practical Suggestions to Improve Sleep

First, make sure your mattress is as comfortable as possible. Many people with CFS and FM use egg-crate mattress pads or memory foam; some buy special beds which allow them to adjust hardness and position for the greatest degree of comfort.

Second, noise and light sensitivity can interfere with sleep. If your spouse snores, moves around in bed a lot, or gets up during the night, your sleep may be disturbed as a result. Understandably, you may be aware of this but choose to continue sleeping in the same bed anyway. Alternatively, sleeping in another bed or in another bedroom may work for you. You might consider a larger bed.

Similarly, fine-tune the smaller details of your sleep routine. Do you fall asleep with the TV on? A sleep timer for the TV can ease this problem. Is the temperature in the room comfortable or does it require some adjustment? Do you watch the clock when you wake up in the middle of the night and worry about how much sleep you have left or how little sleep you've had? If so, turn the clock around or simply don't look at it.

My Sleep Improvement Techniques

Before discovering extended relaxation as an antidote to the usual agony that was my sleep, very occasionally—once or twice a month—I would have a decent night's sleep. During these nights, I drifted in and out of a restful sleep. Typically, these restful nights were followed by pleasant feelings of physical heaviness in the morning. It wasn't clear to me why I only had these pleasant feelings very rarely and I wasn't sure if it was related to why I slept better. Still, most of my nights, I was just mentally and physically restless.

I started doing thirty to sixty minutes of relaxation before bed, sitting in a comfortable chair or lying on a couch with the radio playing softly in the background. When I woke up in the middle of the night (which happened almost every night) and couldn't get back to sleep in thirty minutes, I got out of bed and again did thirty to sixty minutes of relaxation in a soft chair until I felt sleepy. This get-up technique was annoying, but it did help to focus my thoughts on relaxation and sleepiness, rather than the random worries or exciting things that I would normally think about.

After I started this extended relaxation practice, I began to experience the pleasant heavy sensations in my body in the morning, just as I previously had on those rare nights of good sleep. Pleasant heavy sensations are a sign of deep relaxation (see chapter 7 for more information on R-states). I knew this objectively from teaching relaxation techniques for years, but I hadn't previously made the connection between my good sleep and these heavy sensations. In part this was because it had seemed a stretch to think that I could do one hour of relaxation at bedtime and then seven or eight hours later, after a night's sleep, still feel the effects of it. Yet now the connections all seemed to make sense: with one to two hours of relaxation a night, I usually (but not always) got those pleasant feelings of heaviness and restful sleep the following morning.

Cutting Back on Relaxation

An hour of relaxation before bed and an hour of relaxation in the middle of the night when I would wake up improved my sleeping pattern by 50 percent. I was elated. After all, I was desperate to improve my poor sleep and the run-down feelings it added to my illness. But after two weeks of improved sleep, I decided to cut back on the relaxation. After all, who wants to do two hours of relaxation a day if it's not necessary? So I skipped the relaxation practice before bed and did only the middle of the night relaxation. Still I got restful sleep. Clearly two hours weren't necessary for me.

Next, I cut back on the relaxation in the middle of the night. Instead of getting out of bed and doing relaxation exercises for an hour, I now did only a brief relaxation exercise in bed, for fifteen or twenty minutes, just enough to return to sleep. Although this twenty-minute relaxation did get me back to sleep, my sleep wasn't so restful. Once again, I started to feel the morning malaise that follows a poor night's sleep.

The Importance of Relaxation Recordings

Ultimately, I realized that I needed the additional help of an external relaxer to get to sleep without doing hours of self-relaxation. For me, this took the form of audiobooks, including nonscary novels and interesting biographies. Although twenty minutes of self-relaxation wasn't powerful enough to defeat my stressful thoughts, having an audiotape playing *as I drifted to sleep* kept my attention on the tape. Now I regularly fall asleep and get back to sleep using audiotapes—without having to do extensive self-relaxation techniques or out-of-bed breaks during the night.

CHAPTER 9

Step Three: How to Pace ALL of Your Activity—It's More Than You Think

You may believe that you thrive on being involved in innumerable projects. Yet, nonstop activity can be your downfall as well. Fits and starts of activity when symptoms ease may cause you to run out the clock on your energy while ignoring pain and fatigue. The result: relapses, collapses, crashes, and setbacks.

Because you probably feel some desperation to be well, any easing of your illness probably leads you to hope—and maybe even believe— that you're getting better. And so you celebrate good days by doing all of the activities that you'd like to do—but with the unwanted consequence of increased symptoms.

It seems to make sense that when you are feeling better you should do more. If you don't do more, you may feel this signals giving up, resignation, or defeat. However, this kind of mind-set doesn't allow for much flexibility about how to handle your up time. Consider this: a basic tenet of good mental health is that if a particular behavior consistently produces negative results, then it's better to develop alternatives than to simply hope you won't get the same negative result the next time around. Applying this to CFS and FM, if you always exploit your up time by working to exhaustion and then crashing, perhaps it's time to try a different approach. This chapter explores some helpful alternatives to this push-crash cycle.

How More Activity May Increase Pain

People with CFS and FM may ignore even severe symptoms in order to keep going and get more done. A study conducted by psychologist Perry Nicassio and his colleagues (1995) at the University of California at San Diego concluded that ignoring pain and increasing activity ("active coping") in patients with FM may be detrimental:

> Because of the high degree of pain in FM, active coping may be maladaptive if such tendencies cause patients to ignore appropriate limits to their behavior when their pain is already severe. In this regard it is possible that active coping may unwittingly exacerbate muscular and other physiological mechanisms that may contribute to FM pain. Alternatively, intense pain may drive patients to cope actively (do more) in an effort to control the pain, thus contributing to a vicious cycle of pain and dysfunction (1557).

Your Schedule Is More Flexible Than You Think

Before your illness, you probably completed most things with little difficulty—from household activities and taking care of your family to service to others and professional accomplishment. You may still be trying to keep up with your pre-illness activity level, but now you're probably struggling and feeling overextended.

There are always certain things you must do regardless of their effect on your illness, but you probably have more flexibility than you realize to either rearrange your schedule or do your activities in a more energy-conserving manner. Remember: conserving energy can lead to less pain and fatigue. Now, I realize that it can be very hard to slow down or stop what you're doing when you're in the middle of it and want it completed. But realize that your habits are taking a big toll on your illness. Are you willing to try to do things somewhat differently, if the result is feeling better physically and emotionally?

You may feel that doing less—or doing things more gradually— would demonstrate laziness or underachievement. Or you may fear that doing less will somehow reveal how limited you really are—and keep you that way. The opposite is most likely true: if you moderate and pace your activities, you'll replenish your energy levels and lessen your pain and fatigue (although you may feel some frustration at things not being done by your customary schedule). Can pacing lessen the ups and downs of the illness? It can. But it can also do much more. Pacing, in combination with the other improvement techniques explained in this book, can actually lead to reduced illness severity.

Sometimes it's hard to see how the unpredictable fluctuations of CFS and FM have anything to do with lifestyle factors. Illness patterns aren't solely related to lifestyle—clearly, a biological process plays a significant, if yet unknown, role in these illnesses. However, because the role of this biological process is as yet unknown, you're left to modify what you can: your own behavior.

How Pacing Can Work

Do people who pace—or slow down—their activities really experience illness improvements? The short answer is yes. All of the successful behavioral treatment studies in CFS and FM have taught patients to change *how* they do their activities, and pacing is one technique they have used. Furthermore, I know from the people I counsel—and my own experience—that how you do activities is very important.

Collecting Activity Data on Yourself

I have objective data on myself and one other person that demonstrates this. Once a year, for the past three years, I've hooked myself up to a battery-powered pedometer (step counter) for three weeks in order to observe my level of physical activity on a daily basis and record my energy, fatigue, and stress levels. Barbara, a forty-one-year-old friend of mine who also suffers from CFS agreed to do a similar three-week period of data collection with a pedometer once a year.

During the early stages of her illness, Barbara was so afraid of losing her job that she worked even harder than before in order to prove that she could still function at a high level. Because she was terrified of her illness worsening, she constantly tested herself in an effort to prove that she wasn't getting worse. This constant vigilance most likely helped deplete what little energy Barbara had left. (Constant fear can produce fatigue, and although this isn't the abnormal fatigue of CFS, fear-based fatigue will impact CFS fatigue. You may or may not be able to separate the two types of fatigue; regardless, each influences the other and each can increase the other.)

As Barbara's CFS symptoms grew more intense, the quality of her sleep suffered and she became more fearful. Yet three years later she says she has recovered completely. How did this happen? For one thing, after several months of illness, Barbara lost her fear of becoming an invalid. This lessened her need to be constantly active. As she learned to adjust to the illness she moved out of this crisis phase, purging herself of fear and desperation, and learning to use pacing and relaxation techniques instead.

At the beginning of Barbara's illness, the pedometer showed an average daily count of 11,000 steps; three years later, when she had recovered, the daily count settled down to 9,000. This may come as a surprise—you probably expected that people would do more after they've recovered. But, after counseling scores of people with these illnesses, what I see time and again is that those who are high functioning (e.g., working full-time) when they're ill tend to do about the same or somewhat less when they're in an improvement phase.

In Barbara's case, she reduced activities that drained her energy. During the early stages of her illness, she worked a fifty-hour week, plus exhibited her nature photography (a hobby of hers) all over the country. Now, in a recovery phase, Barbara worked fewer hours and spent less time away from home at these exhibitions—which, although exciting, were also very energy-depleting. For Barbara, activity reductions were clearly beneficial.

In my case, my average daily step count also decreased over a two-year period, from about 9,000 to 7,500. I believe this reduction is one of the reasons I now have less fatigue and more energy. On the other hand, for people who can do very little, activity reduction is probably not an appropriate solution. See the following sections for more information.

Pace Everything You Do

Pacing should be applied to any and all of your activities— whether physical and mental—that are potentially exhausting. The first thing to do is to review your daily activities and note which ones produce significant symptom flare-ups. Keep a daily log of your activities and rate your fatigue and pain levels (on a 0–10 scale) before and after each activity. Then examine your symptom-worsening activities and see if you can break them up into smaller units or pieces.

Now, I recognize that you have certain obligations, certain things you must do, that will increase your symptoms and stress level. Even so, you can still figure out ways to address these obligations that are less stressful and more connected to feelings of calm (rather than pressure and aggravation). The following are some pacing suggestions that will help you accomplish this.

You can pace mental activities, particularly those that require the focusing of your attention (this might include such things as social conversations, phone calls, balancing a checkbook, and so forth), by breaking them into smaller chunks and spreading them out. For instance, you can space out your phone calls, especially those that involve intense conversations. If you still feel your energy declining, you can shorten the calls themselves. Remember: getting things done according to some ideal schedule isn't as important as getting things done in a less exhausting way.

For physical activities, spread out the routine errands, chores, and other responsibilities that drain your limited resources. When time permits, schedule a healing morning or afternoon—a substantial chunk of time during which you devote all, or nearly all, of your energies to relaxation and pleasurable experiences. This will refresh you both mentally and physically.

On good days, when energy returns, it can be extraordinarily difficult to hold yourself back from diving into things. A good rule of thumb is to do the activity you want to do, but do it at a much slower speed or with significantly less intensely. You may not get the satisfaction of doing it all completely at one time, but you will gain the ability to sustain your effort long term. (To achieve just this level of improvement can make me enthusiastic.)

Pacing helps you to level out your daily activities so that on relatively bad days you can keep to your schedule rather than significantly reducing it; and similarly, on good days, you can keep to your schedule rather than substantially increasing it. I realize these principles are not easily accepted, but they work better than any other system that I am aware of. This technique of leveling out activities, on a day-to-day basis, has been found to be very successful in CFS and FM in behavioral treatment studies.

■ Elizabeth's Story: An Example of Pacing

Elizabeth, at fifty-one, had had CFS for twenty years. She had been widowed for five years and had four grown children. Her symptom checklist indicated severe mental and physical fatigue, memory and concentration problems, post-exertional malaise, and shortness of breath from minor activity. Although she was unable to work because of her illness, she was generally a happy person.

She described herself as being compulsively neat, which was expressed through hurried, energy-draining housework. Activity records showed that Elizabeth did several hours of housework every day, especially cleaning, straightening, and laundry. Her energy was depleted by this massive push to make her house look nice. As a result, she would collapse from fatigue about once a week. Prior to a collapse, her head would hurt, but rather than slow down once she got this signal, Elizabeth would hurry to finish her chores before the crash came.

To change this push-crash pattern, Elizabeth was first asked to do something small but very difficult for her: leave the house without making her bed, something she had never done before. She feared that doing this would make her a bad housekeeper, an almost ruinous self-evaluation for her. But she was able to do it. By session three, she had developed a much less hurried attitude about getting the housework done and was able to let other things go undone as well. She now paced her housework, so that chores were broken down into smaller steps and done gradually rather than in a single exhausting effort. As she very aptly said, "I don't want to be a slave to my house if it hurts me."

By her fifth and final session, Elizabeth was feeling much better physically and emotionally; she had realized that putting too many activities too close together was a problem for her. Breaking up the housework into more manageable portions was an important first step toward illness improvement.

■ Jim's Story: Pace Even When You Can Do Very Little

Jim, one of the people I counseled who was housebound with CFS, did a masterful job of pacing various activities during the day, from eating to walking. However, Jim viewed paperwork in a different category, one exempt from pacing. Rather than complete a written application in a measured way—perhaps by completing one question at a time and resting in between—Jim would furiously do the entire application in one sitting. This increased his mental confusion and physical fatigue.

Jim had always prided himself on doing paperwork efficiently and expeditiously—completing paperwork tasks all at once reflected his personal values about accomplishment. He didn't even consider pacing his paperwork; his value system simply wouldn't allow it. As a result, Jim would put off any paperwork until he felt well enough to complete an entire paperwork task at one time. (This is a small-scale version of the overwork-collapse pattern so common in CFS and FM.)

When Jim finally applied the pacing concept to his paperwork, although he had to spread the task out over several days, he finished it without any symptom-worsening.

So, examine your daily activities and identify those that exhaust you the most; apply pacing to these exhausting activities first. You'll soon see the difference: less concentrated effort means less impact on your illness.

Pacing as a Major Lifestyle Change

After you've starting pacing your most exhausting activities, consider making the pacing of all of your daily activities your ultimate goal. If you choose to progress toward this goal, you'll begin to modify longstanding hyperactive patterns—e.g., eating fast, walking fast, and talking at high speed. The underlying philosophy of hyperactivity could be stated as follows: "Everything I do must be productive, efficient, and purposeful. Nothing must be left undone." Daily pacing, however, frees you from this frenetic pursuit of accomplishments, large and small. Pacing will save you energy and if it's done thoroughly, over time you'll have *more* energy. (You may have liked your old fast and furious lifestyle, but your body is now telling you that your demands on it have exceeded its capacity; respect these messages from your body.)

■ Elaine's Story: How Pacing Can Help

Elaine, at forty-one, had been ill with FM for ten years. Her condition left her highly stressed and unable to work. An ongoing family conflict about care for her aging parents was also disturbing her deeply. Despite these ongoing problems, she was able to benefit from attending an FM illness-management group: she learned stress reduction and pacing techniques that helped to reduce her high level of stress and pain. She also participated in a warm-water pool therapy program, doing gentle stretching and mild aerobics. After her pool therapy sessions, Elaine would feel so good that she was tempted to immediately jump into a number of home improvement projects.

However, she wisely resisted this temptation and paced her schedule instead. For example, she limited herself to a reasonable fifteen minutes of garage cleaning at a time as opposed to a pain-producing, one-hour commitment. To cope with these reduced fifteen-minute work periods, Elaine would think to herself, "It's not perfect, but it's okay." This belief helped her to reduce the entrenched perfectionism that had previously made it difficult to do things in a healthier way.

Here are some additional ideas about how you can pace a variety of activities:

Eating—eat more slowly; enjoy every bite of your food; eat with a sense of enjoyment and restful contemplation.

Walking—walk more slowly and easily; there's no rush.

Speaking—measure your words; speaking quickly can be mentally and physically draining.

Housecleaning—consider spreading cleaning tasks over several days; you may hate to look at an unorganized house, but is a massive one-time effort worth the exhaustion that follows?

Working—take short relaxation breaks regularly (thirty to sixty seconds) to calmly focus on your breathing; this will renew and refresh you, and may give you greater mental clarity as well. (This is pacing via brief pauses for relaxation.)

Socializing—limit interactions to a few minutes at a time; tell those you are with that you tire easily; turn down social invitations if they require more commitment than your energy level allows.

Now, I'm not suggesting that you're doing *all* of these activities at breakneck speed, but you're probably doing at least some of them much more rapidly than you need to. To move toward wellness, you need to make self-care important. This is a gradual process, which requires a series of choices and decisions that may seem to violate your view of yourself. However, part of the reason that you're ill is because what you think is good for you isn't actually working for you in practice! Yes, it would be nice if people with CFS and FM were so constitutionally strong that they could do whatever they wanted without any bad consequence to themselves. But none of us are superhuman. I once saw a bumper sticker that read:

I AM WOMAN

I AM INVINCIBLE

I AM TIRED

This should ring a bell. It's time to stop ringing it.

■ Nancy's Story: Pacing in a High-Functioning Individual with FM

Nancy, a thirty-seven-year-old schoolteacher and mother of three, had a long-standing case of FM—and a particularly hectic schedule. In addition to full-time teaching, Nancy ran educational programs at her church and was a part-time musician, playing both clarinet and piano in a community orchestra. She worried a great deal, both about her kids and about completing her daily schedule. Covering all the bases and doing everything right were so important to her that she often obsessed about not being thoroughly prepared.

Nancy regularly experienced severe pain in her shoulders and neck. Although this pain could be alleviated for several hours with medication, it would then return, often waking her up at night. She also noticed pain flares during certain activities, such as long phone conversations; pain would also often increase when she was in between activities rather than in the midst of doing them. Her pain was unbearable—but at the same time, Nancy didn't like the idea that she had to take medication in order to get relief.

Nancy had seen numerous doctors and tried interventions from physical therapy to pain patches without results. Because medication worked to some extent, I certainly did not want to minimize its benefits. Yet, it appeared that lifestyle and stress factors played a significant role in her pain. If my evaluation was correct, then long-term, lifestyle change and stress reduction were essential for sustained improvement.

Initially, I had Nancy keep an activity and stress record for one week. This record revealed a pattern of rushing and planning throughout the day, so the next step was to get her to begin to question her behavior at key moments during the day. For example, she was to ask herself, "Do I need to be rushed right now?" If possible, she would then let herself slow down. Similarly, throughout her day she was to ask herself,

"Do I need a break right now?" and remind herself, "I don't have to get there as fast as I can."

Nancy also had trouble in the beginning with relaxation exercises because she would find herself thinking, "What did I forget to do?" whenever she attempted to relax. However, as she began to respond positively to relaxation sessions, she was able to slow down her activities and enjoy the easier pace. She no longer felt that she had to fill up her time with more activity just for the sake of it. Instead, she now allowed herself to take breaks, such as calmly sitting down for twenty minutes with a cup of tea. Also, by doing relaxation exercises at bedtime with greater focus and less worry, Nancy was no longer waking up in the middle of the night with pain that required additional medication. And as her pain receded, it changed from being sharp and oppressive to merely dull and tolerable.

In only four sessions Nancy reported 25 percent less pain (with less pain medication) and 50 percent less stress—a good start on the improvement/recovery path. Because she was willing to maintain her restructured lifestyle, she could continue to expect—if not complete recovery given the biological aspects of the illness—certainly a level of improvement far better than her presenting condition.

■ Christa's Story: Pacing in a Nine-Year-Old with CFS

Christa, a nine-year-old girl with severe CFS, required a home tutor because she could only attend school every two or three weeks, and only for a day or two at a time. When she did go to school, Christa could attend classes for three to four hours, but then felt so tired and headachy that she had to return home.

After consulting with her mother, I put Christa's school attendance on a pacing schedule. It began with attendance every day—but for only one morning class. Christa was then told to come home, rather than risk a collapse from staying longer. She fiercely resisted this plan because she wanted the option to stay in school longer if she felt she could handle it. (Sounds just like adults with CFS, doesn't it?) But finally, with her mother's persuasion and support, the new schedule was agreed upon.

To Christa's complete surprise, she was able to go to that single morning class every day without any problems. However, she still stubbornly insisted that she should be able to stay for a second class if she had enough energy to do so. I explained to her that, without a steady and gradual increase in her school time, she would simply revert to her old pattern: using up all of her energy when she had it and then suffering weeks of downtime. With her mother's support, the new pacing schedule was maintained and gradually increased—and by the end of the following month, Christa was able to resume full-time attendance.

I should mention that stress factors played a significant role in Christa's illness. In particular, she had a strained— and possibly verbally abusive—relationship with her father, although he wasn't directly involved with her after her parent's divorce. This is typical in many cases of CFS and FM: both the immediate stresses of the illness and larger life stressors, such as family and work pressures, have a major impact on the severity of the condition.

Although I'm a firm believer in pacing daily activities, both physical and mental, I never realized until more recently that sometimes, pacing needs to be done on a very minimal level indeed. Michael's story demonstrates how even the smallest of changes can be important steps on the road to improvement.

■ Michael's Story: A Bedridden Patient Slowly Improves

Michael, a forty-nine-year-old physician ill with CFS for a year, punctuated his daily rest with structured activities, including brushing his teeth, eating, bathing, and light reading. This may not sound like a lot, but this schedule was actually a significant improvement over his previously bedridden state. (Both Michael's structured activities and his daily schedule itself are forms of pacing. As with pacing a single activity over many days, a daily schedule should be maintained regardless of illness fluctuations; regular habits will be lost if the person breaks the schedule when feeling better or succumbs to the illness when feeling worse.)

I recommended that Michael begin a one-minute exercise schedule: thirty seconds of stretching in the morning and thirty seconds of stretching in the afternoon. He protested that this was a ridiculously small amount of time and couldn't possibly do any good. He tried to bargain with me about the schedule: "Well, if I do the thirty seconds and I still feel okay, I want to go on then for another minute or two." (This is how you get into trouble: by ignoring pacing and going the distance—even when the distance is "only" two minutes of exercise.) When I explained to him that this type of program had been very successful in a behavioral treatment study, he agreed to give it a try, but remained skeptical.

Michael practiced this stretching program for the next several weeks. In the beginning, he could only do the exercise in the afternoon when energy permitted. By the end of the several week period, however, he could do the exercises in both the morning and the afternoon. His range of motion improved and he increased his time from thirty to sixty seconds.

Michael was surprised by these positive results. In the past, he would have dismissed such minimal improvements, but now he viewed it as a hopeful sign: he had attained a level of control over his physical activity that he hadn't previously had. And this improved ability was achieved through his *own* efforts.

Pace Even When You're Feeling Better

It's most important to continue pacing your activity even when you are feeling better, only at a somewhat higher level. Strongly resist the temptation to make up for lost time or finish tasks without regard to their effect on you. Pacing means taking control of your activity and downshifting the tendency to do too much. When you overdo activity, you as a rational being are not really in charge; your perfectionism and must-do work ethic take over and subdue your rational self. Attempting to push yourself to your desired activity level is both self-defeating and detrimental to your health. Perhaps most importantly, it also just doesn't work over the long run. How many times do you want to repeat this same self-defeating activity and get the same negative result? Moderating your activity makes sense; in addition to its long-term health benefits (reduced fatigue and pain), it will restore your feeling of control over your life.

CHAPTER 10

Step Four: Identifying and Lessening Anger

There are any number of understandable reasons to be angry when you have CFS and FM. In people with FM, self-anger seems to be the most common form of anger. In people with CFS, anger is more likely to be directed outward, toward dismissive physicians, unsupportive family and friends, and any others who express skepticism or even ridicule about the existence of the illness. People with FM are much more likely to suppress their anger than people with CFS, although they may be aware of their anger toward themselves.

Anger is normal in this situation—almost anyone would be angry and frustrated by a sudden chronic illness that cannot be overcome or controlled; self-anger can easily arise when you find that you can't do all you want to do and as a result your efforts fall well below your normal high standards of accomplishment. You may also experience anger-provoking thoughts, such as, "I should be able to control this illness!" Or, "My inability to control this illness makes me weak and useless." Or, "If I'm not busy helping others, people will think I'm not good."

When you were well, anger was much easier to cover up. Why? Because you could do more. Then, it was much easier to get totally immersed in an activity and distract yourself from anger, self-doubt, a sense of inferiority, or feelings of badness. Getting involved in meaningful activities was probably a lifeline for you to greater feelings of self-worth; then, busyness was probably a rapid-fire (albeit temporary) way to overcome frustration at things being left undone.

A Published Anger List

A study done at the University of Washington in Seattle (Okifuji, Turk, and Curran 1999) produced the following list of things that chronic pain patients were most angry about. Topping the list, 74 percent said they were angry at themselves, while 62 percent were angry with their health care providers.

Most Frequent Anger Targets for Chronic Pain Patients

1. Self

2. Health care providers

3. Significant other

4. Whole world

5. Person who caused injury

6. Insurance company

7. Attorney

8. God/Destiny

It's very easy to understand feelings of anger toward health care providers. Often, health care providers don't understand your symptoms or aren't able to treat them; if in addition, a provider indicates disbelief or skepticism about your illness, this rejection can escalate already high levels of stress and demoralization.

Although the opening of the Hippocratic oath is "First, do no harm ... ," harm is clearly done when an illness is pronounced a non-entity or a trivial self-inflicted psychological problem by your health care provider. Advice given by doctors can be just as infuriating—it can range from "do volunteer work" to "eat less chocolate." So anger at doctors and other health care providers is quite understandable.

Of course, skepticism and disbelief can also extend to family members and friends. They may be deceived by the healthy appearance of the person with CFS and/or FM, and baffled by the ups and downs of an illness that allows you to be functional one day only to be in bed the next. To the people close to you, these dramatic changes may seem like voluntary choices rather than unpredictable fluctuations in your condition. Again, you may react to this skepticism and disbelief with anger and hurt.

The Difficulty in Identifying Emotions: How This Can Affect You

A good number of people with these illnesses—particularly those with FM—have difficulty identifying their negative feelings, most commonly anger and hurt. For instance, if you have an encounter with another person where you feel slighted or demeaned in some way, you may not immediately be aware of these feelings. It may not be until a few minutes—or hours—later that you identify these negative feelings and allow yourself to feel angry or hurt about what happened. Or you may not even get that far—even days later you may still be unaware of this hidden anger; it will, however, be festering internally.

■ Mary's Story: An Example of Hidden Anger

At forty-eight, Mary was diagnosed with FM; her particular case involved widespread pain, flu-like symptoms, chronic infections, severe fatigue, and concentration and memory difficulties. Her daily activities included low-level cleaning, watching TV, and some limited socializing. Mary felt very angry with herself for being so weak and inactive, but at the same time, she found it almost impossible to say she was angry at anyone else about anything. For example, she was uncomfortable openly expressing anger about a traumatic incident at her previous job in which she was physically harassed by a supervisor. She would speak in a way that suggested anger but would deny the anger itself. When asked about this, she said that being angry at others violated her image of herself as a nice person.

Studies of Hidden Anger

This difficulty in identifying and expressing negative feelings contributes to the stress, pain, and fatigue that you experience. Several studies have confirmed this connection. Perhaps the most impressive evidence comes from a study done by psychologist Melanie Greenberg and her associates (1999). Greenberg and colleagues studied ninety-three patients with FM over a two-year period. She found that those patients who had the greatest difficulty in *identifying* and *expressing* their negative emotions at the beginning of the study suffered greater levels of pain and disability two years later—regardless of the patient's initial level of pain and disability. It seems likely that the stress of pent-up emotions in these individuals may have contributed to their pain and disability.

Studies of chronic pain also point to a relationship between anger and illness severity. One study, conducted by Dr. Robert Kerns and his colleagues (1994) at the West Haven VA Medical Center in Connecticut, found a link between unexpressed anger and pain intensity in people with chronic pain. Other studies have found that chronic pain patients have less awareness of personal anger when compared to other medical patients. Also, chronic pain patients show greater anger suppression compared to healthy control subjects.

Some researchers have suggested that suppressing negative emotions—particularly anger—may increase an individual's pain sensitivity by lowering the body's natural levels of *endorphins* (morphine-like substances that alleviate pain). Alternatively, increased pain sensitivity may be triggered by increased muscle tension at the site of pain.

This problem with anger recognition often directly contributes to the conflicts people with CFS and FM have in relationships. However, when people with these illnesses become more aware of their feelings and learn to express them more freely, they then feel more empowered, less stressed—and often less ill.

The Difficulty in Expressing Negative Emotions

In addition to a difficulty in recognizing anger, people with CFS and FM may also have great difficulty openly expressing personal feelings about what they do and do not want. In one early study (Dailey et al. 1990) that compared people with FM to people with rheumatoid arthritis and healthy controls, 57 percent of the FM patients endorsed "inability to express yourself" as a significant daily hassle, while only 10 percent of the arthritis patients and 36 percent of the healthy controls agreed with this statement. A similar pattern was found with another statement, "fear of confrontation"—this one was endorsed as a daily stress by 43 percent of the FM patients but only 10 percent of the arthritis patients and 14 percent of the healthy control participants.

Why do people with CFS and FM have such difficulty expressing their personal feelings, especially negative ones? Several factors are probably in play:

A Desire to Be Viewed as Good

This is the need to be viewed as the good little girl or boy who never makes waves or inconveniences people. You may fear that if you do voice complaints, others will view you as a bad person. For example, "If I complain to my spouse, friends, or anyone else, they'll think less of me." Or, "I can't handle the idea of people not liking me."

No Right to Complain

The belief that you do not have the right to complain is based on the perception of your life as pretty good—or at least not so bad. For example, "Who am I to complain? After all, I have a good husband and nice kids, a nice home . . ."

A Fear of Selfishness

This is the fear that complaints are nothing more than selfish out-bursts. You may believe that any complaining at all shows that you are *not* a well-adjusted independent person who can help everyone without needing anything in return.

Complaints Are for the Weak

This attitude is based on the notion that complaining reveals a personal weakness or an inability to solve your own problems.

The Damage Caused by Holding Back Feelings

You may recognize one or more of these factors above as an important motivating force in your life. You certainly have the right to hold these beliefs, but understand that these fear-based attitudes will have persistent and damaging effects on your mental and physical health. Why? Because you're seeking to do the impossible: to have everyone love, admire, and respect you at all times, while at the same time denying your own needs for support and personal time. You can't win with these core beliefs—no matter how much you do for others, it will never be enough to fulfill all of your own personal needs.

With these do-everything-and-don't-complain beliefs, your self-esteem is also almost entirely based on constant high performance. Anything less will remind you that you aren't good enough. And despite denying your own needs, you'll still feel the ache and depriva-tion of not having these needs fulfilled. The idea of being self-sufficient isn't the problem; the problem is the unrealistic goal of becoming so independent that you need nothing and no one. This is a denial of your humanity.

The greater the suppression of your most important desires and feelings (particularly anger), the more stress, pain, and fatigue you're likely to have. Again, it's not my intention to reduce CFS and FM to disorders of stress; however, I do firmly believe that these stressful, pent-up feelings and desires play an important role in the severity of your illness.

How to Better Identify Your Negative Feelings

Now that we have explored why people with CFS and FM have difficulty expressing negative emotions, let's examine what people are so angry about. Because anger, hurt, and disappointment are often hidden just below the conscious level, you may not be aware of these emotions, but with some practice, you can learn to identify them.

For many people with these illnesses, this hidden anger is fueled by unmet expectations of support and encouragement from others. Ask yourself: what are the expectations that I have of my spouse, children, friends, doctors, and others in general? Next ask yourself: to what extent have these individuals failed my expectations and disappointed me? And: what emotions do I feel about these disappointments? I would doubt that you feel only mild disappointment, that you just calmly think, "Oh, it's too bad that other people don't provide me with much support, encouragement, or caring." Unless you are shockingly rational about the lack of support from others, you will almost certainly experience some level of frustration, distress, and anger. Try to acknowledge your right to feel that anger. If you can accomplish this first step, you can then do something useful with your emotions.

If you're ready to become more aware of your feelings, I suggest that you begin by logging your feelings whenever you have encounters with other people that leave you stressed or upset. First, write down what was discussed; then, ask yourself if you feel angry, hurt, anxious, guilty, and/or frustrated. Focus on these emotions as best you can—it may be difficult. Next, focus on the beliefs and thoughts related to these emotions. These thoughts and beliefs usually contain should's and must's and ought to's either directed at yourself or the other person. Write down both these thoughts and the emotions that are related to them. Here are some examples:

Thoughts: "They know how busy I am. How dare she ask me to do that?!"

Feelings: Anger, frustration, hurt, disappointment.

Thoughts: "She seemed to be cross with me. What did I do to create that? I've got to get her on my good side again."

Feelings: Anxiety, guilt.

Thoughts: "I do so much for him. He gives me no support. Doesn't he realize this? I think he should."

Feelings: Anger, hurt.

Give yourself the right to have these feelings. Again, they are part of your humanity.

How to Better Express Negative Feelings

Next, give yourself permission to express these feelings to others. Write down an assertive, yet tactful answer to a particular person—or to people in general—for when you feel some sense of disapproval or rejection. Practice your assertiveness in front of the mirror. Practice for your next encounter—this could be with your spouse, whom you might want more support from, or perhaps a neighbor or a person at a PTA meeting or a member of your church with a demand on your time. Recognize that you have a personal feeling niggling at you about their requests.

When you do actually assert yourself, give yourself both the right to your feelings and the right to personal time. You may experience mixed feelings during these assertive exercises—possibly at every step of the way—because this level of forwardness may seem to conflict with the person that you wish to be. But remember: that person, who strives to be all things to all people, is also an overstressed, overburdened, and—at the core—unhappy person. Reducing the unnecessary responsibilities that stress and exhaust you will help free up the time you need to take care of yourself—and open up the opportunity to feel better, physically and emotionally.

Your Right to Express What You Feel

These statements, when read and practiced on a daily basis, will help reinforce your belief in your right to express your feelings:

- I have the right to complain about something that is important to me.

- I have the right to be discontent, even if my circumstances are generally good.

- I have the right to ask for help and support.

- I have the right to feel hurt and angry.

- I have the right to say no.

- I may like helping and pleasing others, but I don't have to.

- I am an adult now, not a child. Expressing myself is the adult thing to do.

Now, the downside of this greater expressiveness may well be that others do not continue to view you as the all-helpful, always good superperson. This is the trade-off you must consider: is illness improvement worth the risk that others may no longer view you as Ms./Mr. Nice because you now (sometimes) question or say no to a request? It's up to you. This isn't an easy choice—if it were, you would have made it long ago.

Your right to express negative feelings extends to family, friends, doctors, or whoever has disappointed you for whatever reasons. This is your right. There are risks in doing this; for one thing, people may not be comfortable with your new ability to express negative feelings. But why should they be? They may also react with surprise if they are accustomed to your unflappably cheerful and agreeable personality. This is also to be expected. However—and more importantly—if you express your concerns and ask for what you really want, whether it be support or relief or respect in whatever form, you may be surprised. When you ask for something you want, you may just get it, at least to some degree.

Because asking for what you want or don't want may be a relatively new experience to you, I suggest you start your assertive statements thus: "I would like . . . (more support, more help, etc)." Or, "I would rather not . . . (volunteer, do extra work, etc.)." Or, "I don't like . . . (what you said, what you did, etc.)." If you feel a temptation to blast someone with pent-up anger, try to control that temptation and express your intense feelings more constructively using the ideas above. If you're very angry, say so without the blast—this approach is much more likely to get a better reception from the person you're talking to.

■ Nancy's Story: An Example of Voicing Personal Feelings

At fifty-nine, Nancy had had CFS for five years. During her counseling sessions, she had begun to realize that outings with friends could be very draining and exhausting if they went on for too long. But she felt she couldn't leave early. Wouldn't this hurt her friends and make her look selfish and uncaring of their needs? Finally, after recognizing how much this extra time with her friends was actually hurting her, she began to allow herself to decline invitations and leave outings before her friends did. This required some degree of assertiveness training, but now, Nancy leaves her friends before exhaustion sets in, and she feels refreshed by these outings, rather than worn out. "They can handle my leaving early," says Nancy.

What to Tell Yourself

The following self-assertive statements will help you believe the new ideas introduced above. Review all of these coping statements, identifying the ones that are most effective for you—then practice them for five minutes a day (a pretty minimal investment that will yield major benefits to your well-being, stress level, and pain severity).

- ■ I can balance my personal needs with those of others.

- ■ I do not need to completely sacrifice myself for others.

- ■ It is unrealistic to think that I can solve all of my own problems; this kind of overreaching only causes me more stress—and solves little.

- ■ I will feel guilty whether or not I ask for more support, so why not ask?

- ■ When I put aside my need to be completely independent at all times, I realize that a more supportive relationship with my family and friends is something I both want and have a right to.

Let's face it: sometimes you won't be liked or loved—or feel good about yourself—when you express an objection or a complaint or even a simple request. It's still important, however, for both your health and your self that you be assertive in taking care of your personal needs. To cope with these potential reactions, practice these additional self-statements:

- Fulfilling my own needs will lead to a more balanced, flexible life, a life that does not have to be completely dominated by others' approval of my goodness.

- The goal of total goodness and complete approval from others is unrealistic and unachievable.

As you express negative emotions and reduce your need to be viewed as good, you'll begin to feel some level of relief. Also, with greater assertiveness of your own needs, you'll start to get more of what you want from your family, friends, and doctors. There's no guarantee, of course, but until you start making such requests, no one can know what you really need from them.

Self-Anger: How to Stop Persistent Self-Criticism

Self-condemnation doesn't motivate—it only produces useless stress and self-anger. One way to avoid self-condemnation is by learning not to equate your *self* with every action that you do or don't do. By practicing the following coping statements for only five minutes a day, you can begin to rethink your view of yourself:

- I am not equal to my limitations. I can appreciate whatever activity or involvement is possible for me—and regret what I cannot do—but I do not need to berate myself.

- I do not have to rate myself as a person based on every action I take.

- Expressing a complaint does not make me a bad person—it only shows that I am a human being with legitimate needs.

Reducing Anger with More Realistic Expectations

Expressing negative emotions can also be the first step toward examining the unmet expectations you have for others and yourself. The goal is to have realistic expectations—then anger and other negative feelings will diminish and your stress-related symptoms will become less severe.

What are realistic expectations? First, I would suggest minimizing expectations altogether. Expectations are implicit demands that others behave in a certain way. Of course, everyone develops expectations for others—there's nothing criminal about them. But if others don't live up to your expectations, it's better to feel that this is only unfortunate or inconvenient, not devastating. For instance, a study of marriages found that partner satisfaction in long-lasting marriages increased after twenty years—not because husbands and wives became better husbands and wives, but because old expectations about how the other spouse should behave were dropped.

Your expectations may extend to doctors who are "supposed to" try to help you. But as you may have discovered, doctors aren't always helpful. For a number of reasons, doctors may simply express disbelief rather than try to understand your condition. Although anger at such disbelief is understandable, it's better to counteract your anger with statements such as, "I can't convince anyone I am ill who doesn't want to believe it." And, "Their disbelief doesn't negate the reality of my illness."

I do believe that anger and other stressful emotions play a role in making your illness as severe as it is and that alleviating these stressors will lessen symptoms, sometimes to a large degree.

CHAPTER 11

Step Five: Finding Relief from Worry, Discouragement, and Guilt

People suffering from CFS or FM may experience a variety of jarring negative emotions—including anger, grief, discouragement, worry, and guilt. Coping with the emotions of grief, discouragement, worry, and guilt (anger has its own special chapter because it's so important—see chapter 10) can not only help improve your day-to-day well-being, it can also aid in your overall improvement—particularly when these coping skills are well-learned. And without the burden of these negative emotions, you'll have a greater chance to enjoy positive feelings.

Grieving Illness Losses

Acknowledging the losses you experience when you're ill is a healthy and important process—a process that sets the stage for future healing. Writing down these losses and your feelings about them is one way to begin this process. As an unidentified woman with disabling CFS wrote on a Web site:

> I miss my family life and the identity I got from it. My limitations now make it difficult to see myself as valuable in relation to others. And that perception of being less than what I was is transmitted to others—they see me as less. Trying to create a new sense of self with the limited resources that I still do have is very disturbing and difficult, perhaps because I feel so desperate to find that new meaning and identity. I wish this problem would be more often discussed in the CFS community. I do believe that a new sense of self can be created. Helping people understand how to live with impairments would be an important contribution. Or a constructive rethinking of lives that feel diminished. Yes, it is a struggle to create a sense of relevance and usefulness in life when one's beliefs about living a worthwhile life have been centered so much around helping others—but it can be done.

Discouragement

Discouragement is often the natural result of illness symptoms and limitations, because these limitations often lead to a reduced sense of purpose. Discouragement is also one of those emotions that can intensify the all-encompassing malaise of your illness, a malaise that dampens your desire and enthusiasm. Persistent discouragement will imperceptibly meld into your illness experience and further reduce your quality of life; moreover, your illness will seem much worse to you if you concentrate your attention on your feelings of discouragement.

While it's good to recognize feelings of discouragement, it's not healthy to dwell on them. If you find yourself getting preoccupied with all the negative things in your life now that you are ill, it's best to take a step back. Yes, you do have the illness and its limitations, but dwelling on these things requires *thinking*. This type of thinking can be changed.

To change your discouragement-related negative thinking patterns, first identify your negative thoughts (e.g., "I'm so sick, I'm so sick, I'm so sick!" or "I can't stand this!"). Then, refocus on what you *can* do. Appreciate the rewards and good feelings that follow from accomplishments, however small these accomplishments may seem compared to your preillness activities.

Jim, a patient with CFS who successfully let go of his feelings of discouragement, described the transformation of his thinking patterns thus:

> *When I'd been ill for eighteen months I could still work part-time, but every day seemed like a struggle. I couldn't do my exercise. I didn't have the good feelings I used to have. I wondered if I would ever be well again. This type of thinking continued for many months. But eventually I realized that my illness was worsened by thinking these demoralizing thoughts. I was dwelling on all the negatives—and feeling worse as a result. Yes, my CFS was a problem, but it didn't have to totally dominate my life.*
>
> *Rather than focusing on how compromised I was with this illness, I began to give myself credit for what I could do and I began to experiment with doing new, low-effort activities that might make me feel better. This started with very low-level walking—five minutes a day. To my surprise, it really helped. Understanding how my feelings of discouragement affected me was an important first step in actively challenging my negative thinking and changing my life in small but positive ways.*

Worry

For many people with CFS and FM, worry is also a natural reaction—particularly when new symptoms seem to signal a health crisis. Also, just the thought of future disability can understandably cause worries about the financial necessities of day-to-day living; it's very easy to get immersed in worries that you may never get well again.

Although worry may be automatic for many people with CFS and FM, it's an emotion that can be controlled. Worry doesn't solve problems; it only perpetuates stress. Worrying isn't equivalent to caring about yourself or anyone else—it's merely a repetitive thought process without a constructive end.

One way to diffuse worry is to practice worry-reducing statements such as:

Worrying about my symptoms will not give me any control over what happens. Instead of worrying, I can make a plan about how to deal with my symptoms and my life. This will ease my fears and help me focus on the practical things I can do. Whatever the worst is that might happen—whether unemployment, disability, or difficult relationships—these add up only to unfortunate outcomes, not disasters.

I know—it sounds good on paper, but could you ever really be that calm and rational about a major life crisis? You don't have to become 100 percent rational about your illness, you just need to reduce your worrying as much as possible. Practice worry-reducing thoughts. Start by just reading and rereading the above paragraph for five minutes a day. Even this brief interruption in your daily worry patterns may be enough to take the punch out of the "what if's" and "oh my God!'s" that plague your thoughts.

Guilt

You probably experienced large doses of guilt even before you became ill. If you hold yourself to perfectionistic high standards—standards that rarely can be reached—the guilt of not doing enough may be a persistent theme in your emotional life. And if your sense of self-worth comes from helping family, friends, and others, *not* helping—or not being able to help—can produce intense feelings of guilt.

This notion that you *should* be able to do more for those other people is a core guilt-producing thought. But this "should statement" is a rule that you've created for yourself, not a law of nature. In reality, there is no rule. Setting up unrealistic standards for yourself may seem to be a laudable, inspirational thing to do, but impossibly high standards only perpetuate guilt and self-condemnation. To help lessen these harmful feelings of guilt, I suggest practicing some personalized variation on the following statements:

- I will do what I can reasonably do, and I will value this achievement rather than condemning myself for what cannot be done.

- Guilt neither makes me do more, nor changes my behavior—it only sustains bad feelings.

It can take considerable practice to rethink your ideas about your personal worth, but it's healthier to define your personal worth not just by what you do for others but also by what you do for yourself. You're entitled to take care of yourself without guilt.

CHAPTER 12

Step Six: Easing into Pleasant Events and Pleasurable Feelings

Pleasant, uplifting feelings naturally arise from certain things you do. However, it's much more difficult to enjoy even simple pleasures when you're ill. Illness can block your attempts to seek out pleasant events and the good feelings normally produced by them. However, the importance of pleasant experiences as an antidote to the burdens of your illness cannot be overstated.

A Study of Pleasant Events and Improvement in CFS

In research on healthy adults, *pleasant mood induction*—imagining or participating in an activity that will lift your mood and create a pleasant emotional state—has produced healthy changes in stress hormones as well as feelings of increased energy, reduced anger, and improved pain tolerance (Brown et al. 1993). These findings can be applied to CFS and FM as well.

A study conducted by Colette Ray et al. (1995) on the positive and negative life events that took place over one year in 130 people with CFS uncovered a very interesting result: those patients who reported the highest number of positive events had significantly lower scores at the end of the year on measures of fatigue, impairment, anxiety, and depression. (Negative life events were correlated with higher anxiety but unrelated to other illness factors.) As the authors of this illuminating study suggest, positive events and experiences can, indeed, make an important contribution to recovery in CFS.

Of course, playing devil's advocate, you could argue that symptom reduction may have occurred first, with pleasant events following afterward as patients became more able to do a greater number of enjoyable things. However, the results of this study are consistent with several others; for example, a study conducted by Patrick Dailey et al. (1990) found that positive daily moods were associated with pain reduction in patients with FM.

Pleasant experiences and moods can lessen illness stress and even improve functioning—sometimes only temporarily, but sometimes for long periods.

The Powerful Effects of a Single Pleasant Experience

I personally experienced a particularly memorable instance of pleasant mood creation one winter day, as I walked with my girlfriend and her six-year-old daughter in a snow-covered forest. New-fallen snow clung to branches and twigs; snow-covered tree limbs arched gracefully over the narrow trail and the sun glinted brilliantly off upper tree branches glazed slick with ice. Before us, the trail was blanketed in white snow, pristine and completely untouched. The quiet stillness of the forest and its breathtaking natural beauty enveloped us. We had captured a unique moment in time—we felt wonder, serenity, transcendence.

These pleasurable feelings lasted for several days. For me, this lingering pleasant mood not only increased my energy level, it even revived my fatigue-dampened sexual desire. To a large degree, my fatigue and tiredness were counteracted simply by the ongoing good feelings evoked by that fantasy-like experience. Yet the experience itself was stunningly simple: a leisurely walk in the woods.

Scheduling Pleasant Experiences

In the CFS and FM stress-management groups I've run, the shared experience and camaraderie of the first session often seems to have a lasting effect. By the second session, group participants often report—to their great surprise—reduced symptoms and improved moods. It seems as if the support they receive from the group has a powerful mood-elevating effect all on its own. (In a way this isn't surprising—for many of these individuals, these group sessions were their first interactions with others who understood their illness.)

If your pleasurable experiences are few and far between these days, it's time to work on restoring them. Start by making a list of ten low-effort pleasant activities—perhaps listening to a captivating speaker, sharing an intimate moment with a spouse or close friend, taking a bath, sitting in a park, watching ducks on a pond, reading an absorbing story, etc. Then, select five of these ten items and schedule them for the coming week. (This strategy applies both to those individuals who are quite disabled with limited choices and to high-functioning individuals who simply don't allow themselves time for leisurely enjoyment.)

Stringing Together Your Pleasant Experiences

You may think that joy flows from wellness—or, to be more exact, that only wellness can bring joy—however, the opposite is also true: joy and pleasant experiences can also lead to increased feelings of wellness. When you do pleasant activities, rate them on two scales from one to ten: a pleasant/joyful experience scale and a wellness scale. (Ten represents the greatest feelings of joy/wellness, while one represents the least.) When you discover this joy-wellness connection in yourself, you may at first think it's only a very temporary effect. However, as you generate more and more pleasant experiences, these experiences will produce feelings of wellness that last for more than just a few hours.

You can even begin to string together your pleasant events, so that the wellness feelings will last for days, weeks, or even longer. My guess is that only occasionally in your life have you had enough day-to-day pleasant experiences to generate a long-standing good mood.

The idea of creating a lifestyle with an abundance of pleasant experiences may seem a difficult—if not impossible—goal. However, when you focus on simple pleasures, it becomes possible to connect large numbers of pleasant events together in short periods of time. And by doing so, you increase the possibilities for improvement and perhaps recovery.

Why Vacations May Not Help

Although vacations may seem an obvious solution—and may, indeed generate positive feelings—they're decidedly *not* a panacea. In fact, for some people with CFS and FM, a vacation may bring little improvement—even a week or two at a pleasant getaway location may have little illness impact.

Why? One reason is that you may take your stress with you: your environment may look like vacationland but your thoughts may still be in a very unrelaxing, plotting-and-scheming mode. You can also create stress on vacations by scheduling too much activity—this is particularly likely to happen if you feel somewhat better and want to take advantage of that.

If long vacations don't reduce your stress, examine what you do on these vacations; make sure that your schedule includes both pleasurable, relaxing activities and calming thoughts to go with them.

■ Connie's Story: Pleasant Experiences vs. Family Obligations

Connie, a forty-one-year-old woman who had had FM and CFS for twelve years, suffered from recurrent infections, flu-like symptoms, generalized body pain, and troubles with memory and concentration. She felt considerable stress concerning her elderly and demanding parents—they both resided in assisted care facilities one hundred miles away but expected her to visit them frequently.

After working hard to challenge her core identity as a good little girl who always listened to and obeyed her parents, Connie was able to shut out—at times—the excessive, all-consuming guilt she felt about her parents' situation. And as she turned her mind away from this preoccupation, she was able to focus on pleasant things when they came along. Previously, even a simple thing like watching TV would seem like an indulgence—and would produce intense feelings of guilt. Now, however, Connie could occasionally watch a good TV program guilt-free, taking her mind off her background stress and losing awareness of any pain for several hours.

CHAPTER 13

Step Seven: Getting Support from Others

Support from others can take many forms. On a physical level, support can involve assistance with daily physical tasks (such as lifting or carrying) or household chores. Sometimes sensitive employers may allow flexible work schedules to accommodate illness flare-ups. On an emotional level, support involves spouses, friends, or significant others providing a nonjudgmental forum for the sick individual to express feelings and reactions to the illness. Emotional support doesn't imply any type of advice, direction, or intervention; the supportive person simply listens uncritically. The most difficult type of support to obtain from others is simple understanding. Some very empathic spouses or close friends can offer this type of support, as can some doctors who specialize in CFS and FM (although doctors are necessarily limited in the time they can spend with patients).

In a study of the impacts of a natural disaster (Lutgendorf et al. 1995), researchers looked at the effects of social support in people with CFS who were directly hit by a hurricane. (In general, an individual's *social support* refers to the availability of other individuals to provide feelings of connection and belonging.) For those who reported high levels of social support, hurricane disruption didn't trigger relapses. On the other hand, for those with low levels of social support, the stress of the hurricane was strongly correlated with the severity of relapse. Other studies of social support in chronic illnesses also suggest that support improves an individual's ability to cope with stress and symptoms.

Minimizing the Effects of Bad Relationships

As important as good relationships are in the improvement process, minimizing the influence of bad relationships is equally important. Any bad relationship that is a major part of your life—whether it be with a spouse, significant other, sibling, or parent—can be detrimental to your healing. Dysfunctional relationships create an array of negative emotions, including anger, hurt, anxiety, guilt, and depression. These emotions will stress your fragile physical being and worsen your symptoms.

■ Rob's Story: How a Bad Relationship Can Affect CFS

After eighteen months of CFS, Rob, a fifty-one-year-old attorney, tired very quickly and could only work a few hours a week. He'd been married for two years, to his second wife. He had expected that his wife would be supportive of him in his time of need. But his wife, who also worked full-time, was quite intolerant of his illness. In her words, she didn't "sign on" for this. She had established her own, independent life, which included physical workouts and social contacts with friends; she didn't want to take care of anyone.

Rob had originally wanted an old-fashioned, domestic wife, someone who would take care of his needs, but when he'd met his wife-to-be, he'd been so attracted to her good looks that he'd rationalized away all potential problems. His illness, however, elevated these problems to a crisis level. Ultimately, they got divorced. After the divorce, Rob began to feel much more energetic. Without the stress, anger, and worry of his unfulfilling relationship to deal with on a daily basis, his chances for improvement rose considerably.

Asking for Support

Unsupportive marriages and relationships don't have to end in divorce or breakups—sometimes, support can be improved simply by asking directly for help from spouses and significant others. However, because you may take pride in your self-sufficiency and your ability to meet the needs of others, you may find it very difficult to ask for help for yourself.

Many people with these illnesses—and particularly those with FM—want support and relief from responsibilities, but want this assistance to be offered to them—they don't want to have to ask for it. Why? Because people with CFS and FM often don't feel justified in asking for more support. This is a paradox of sorts. You think you *should* get help and support—from family, friends, or whomever—but are reluctant to ask for it. (See chapter 10 for more discussion of handling this type of conflict.) As a result, the necessary help isn't offered, leaving the ill person with both a full load of responsibilities and a raft of pent-up frustrations. This continuing exertion and stress may then lead to increased pain and fatigue.

In order to deal with a lack of support, give yourself the right to both your feelings of anger and your desire for more support. Yes, you have responsibilities, but you also have the right to ask for what would help you. There's no guarantee, however, that those close to you will recognize and respond to your needs. It would be nice if they did, but even with the best of intentions, they may not. *You* need to assert your own needs rather than expect others to know what you need. Remember: if you ask for what you want, you just might get it.

If you get a negative response from one person, you might still get a positive response from another. And if you don't get the support you're looking for, you'll still learn something valuable about the limits of support that are available to you.

This quote from a person with CFS highlights just how effective social support can be:

> *I am really quite amazed by the positive impact that just talking to an understanding person has had for me. Although I am almost constantly fatigued, that feeling of being really connected was so enjoyable that it seemed to reduce my symptoms for a day or two afterward. There really is a mind-body connection in this illness. Not that CFS is all in your head, but that your emotions can affect the physical part of this illness.*

What If You Ask but Don't Receive?

You may be concerned that not only will increasing your assertiveness *not* get you the desired result, it may actually make things worse—that, for example, instead of offering you support, your spouse, friend, significant other, or doctor will simply reject or even belittle your requests for help. It's true: there's no guarantee of a good outcome. And, unfortunately, there are many people with CFS and FM who encounter this all the time in their family, professional, and social lives. However, most rejections are based on a lack of understanding of your illness; sometimes, with enough patience on your part, others can come to a better understanding, and rejections can turn into help. Regardless, remember: a rejection of a legitimate request does not in any way negate your right to express it.

If you can't get support directly from the people close to you, go to other sources. These could include support groups, psychotherapists who specialize in chronic illness, online chat rooms, and phone or personal relationships with others who are similarly ill.

One important caveat when pursuing support: if support groups or chat rooms are merely forums for exchanging complaints without any constructive goals, they may not be helpful. Talking about symptoms and emotions is important, but your efforts need to be geared toward strategies that lead to improvements in the quality of your life. Otherwise little will change.

Handling a Lack of Support

Not all husbands, wives, or significant others are capable—or willing—to provide emotional support, despite your best efforts. If this is the case for you, you need to give up the expectation that they give you support. What kind of relationship is that? Perhaps not a very good one, but if it's important to you to stay in the relationship, then it's better to feel disappointed rather than bitter or angry or constantly hurt.

■ Sarah's Story: Letting Go of Expectations

Sarah, at thirty-eight, had had FM for seven years. Her husband showed little concern for her condition and expected her to do all of the household chores as well as work full-time. As a result, she was emotionally at a constant low boil, given her husband's neglect. Her only alternative to being angry, she thought, was not to care about him at all. She believed she had just those two emotional settings: enraged or indifferent. And she wasn't comfortable being indifferent for any length of time.

But there was a third option: letting go of her expectations that her husband should be different than he was and allowing herself to feel disappointed and sad instead of angry. She struggled with these ideas for months, until finally she made some progress. She began to accept that support would only come from others: her parents, siblings, and friends. She felt less anger, and her pain lessened as well.

CHAPTER 14

Changing Your Lifestyle When Change Seems Impossible

People with CFS and FM often experiment with lifestyle adjustments in order to maintain as much functioning as possible; thus, you may believe that you've already done everything within your power to cope with the illness, and that the seven steps cannot fit into your lifestyle. If you believe this—for whatever reason—consider the ideas below; you may find that they can open up some fresh possibilities for positive change.

If You're Doing a Lot . . .

Many people tell me they can't make lifestyle changes because they have too many obligations. Of course, there are certain things you *must* do in order to survive and be a parent to your children and a partner to your spouse. However, most of my suggestions can be done—perhaps at a lower level—even when your life is full and you see no way to change it. For example, relaxation practice can be done at work in thirty-second and one-minute chunks throughout the day—even with your eyes open. Similarly, if you're not sleeping through the night, you can use relaxation techniques when you can't sleep. (After all, what else do you have to do in the middle of the night?)

Similarly, although you may have to work, you can still pace your activities throughout the day. First identify your harried behaviors, then break them down into manageable portions that you can do in a deliberate, stepwise, and relaxed manner. You can also always be more assertive and ask for what you want, regardless of your busy schedule. And by reading coping statements for only five minutes a day, you can reduce your anger, guilt, and worry.

Clearly, the more flexibility you have in your schedule, the easier it will be for you to incorporate these practices into your day. But no matter how locked in you are to your daily obligations, these low-effort strategies can be included—and these practices will make your life less stressful, less frenetic, and less taxing to your health.

If You're Doing Not-So-Much . . .

You may be so disabled by your illness that you're unable to work or do very much. As a result, you may believe that your daily schedule—which takes into account your limitations—cannot be changed without major consequences. Some of the techniques in this book may even seem useless or silly. Practicing relaxation (step one), for instance, may seem to be a unhelpful reduction in your activity rather than a potentially positive step. And pacing yourself especially when you are feeling better may seem silly—why should you hold back then?

Yes, it's difficult to change long-standing habits that seem to work for you (at least to some degree). But using these seven steps will help you even when your activity level is fairly low. How? By structuring positive, uplifting, stress-reducing activities into your day. These new techniques may even lead to a greater tolerance of activity, with less pain and fatigue.

■ Patricia's Story: Improving Functioning When You're Doing Not-So-Much

Patricia, a forty-five-year-old woman disabled with CFS, came to me for counseling. During the first few sessions, all she wanted to talk about was her bad relationships with her family and friends. Because she'd already undergone many years of therapy focused on these relationships, I asked her if she really wanted to focus on these same issues yet again. I also told her that talking about bad relationships wouldn't, in and of itself, improve her illness. She was a bit taken aback, but nonetheless kept her counseling appointments.

Although Patricia had few responsibilities, she regularly pushed herself to do exhausting housework. Moreover, she was involved in damaging relationships with various members of her family; visits with them almost always resulted in Patricia receiving harsh words of disapproval for any help she might offer. Not surprisingly, this left her even more stressed and fatigued. Why did she do all of these energy-draining things? Because she had to prove to herself—every day—that she could still function and help her family.

The program we set up helped her to cut back both on her housework and on her visits to her family. She also began to take leisurely, five-minute walks daily. (This walking was designed to increase her tolerance for physical activity rather than build up her aerobic endurance.) Six weeks later, she began to experience improvement in her illness. Six months later, she was much more relaxed about her daily schedule. When in the past she would have raced through her housework—leaving her in bed, exhausted and in pain—she now did things more slowly. As she herself described it, "I'm not on a rigid schedule anymore; I'm doing things as they come, but I still get things done."

Patricia's attitude also changed—she no longer viewed herself as a lazy, uncaring person if she didn't do the things that would exhaust her. She had made the decision to change her life and feel better.

Become a CFS/FM Scientist

In the spring 2002 edition of the *CFIDS Chronicle*, Bruce Campbell, a psychologist with CFS, described how he became a "CFS scientist" in his efforts to improve his illness. After five years of these efforts, Campbell rated his improvement level at about 90 percent—with 100 percent being completely healthy.

How did he do it? First, Campbell maintained a journal of his activity, energy, and stress levels. As a result, he became very aware of the impact of all of his exertions, whether it be out-of-town travel or a five-minute walk. From this, he determined which activities were most likely to lead to relapses. For example, he discovered that a short walk in the afternoon didn't usually trigger symptom flare-ups for him— although a similar walk in the morning often did. With some experimenting, he found that resting for a certain amount of time before and after he walked in the morning lessened his postexercise symptom flare-ups.

Campbell organized each of his days into chunks of low-level activity, and then very, very gradually increased his activity. His efforts required great discipline and patience—but definitely paid off over time.

You may think that *your* relapses come without warning; however, more often than not, you too can track and identify the things you did that led up to the relapse. Once you are aware of those relapse triggers, you have a choice: are the activities that lead to relapses worth doing? A particular event, like a concert or play or get-together, may be so important to you that it *is* worth the relapse. (Many people with these illnesses choose this trade-off from time to time.) However, if relapses are frequent and disruptive, then these triggers may be helping to maintain your illness at its current severity—and blocking improvement. If you identify and then avoid (as much as possible) your relapse triggers using the techniques described in this book, you'll then begin to see illness improvement.

Getting Assistance

You may decide you want to get additional help from a psychotherapist. (A psychotherapist would normally be a licensed psychologist, social worker, or nurse practitioner; psychiatrists have become medication managers, who do little psychotherapy.) The idea of seeking constructive guidance is a good one—the problem is finding a therapist who understands chronic illness in general, and CFS and FM in particular.

Finding a therapist with interest and expertise in these illnesses can be difficult for two reasons: first, because mind-body interactions are often difficult to identify, many therapists prefer not to see people with CFS and FM; second, many psychologists are still quite skeptical about the existence of these conditions. In one seminar on CFS that I presented, a show of hands revealed that roughly half of my audience of professional psychotherapists didn't even believe in the illness. (Why were they at the seminar? They needed the continuing education credits to keep their licenses current.) So finding the right professional can be quite difficult. Try asking your local support-group leader for recommendations; they often know specific therapists who help people with these types of illnesses.

When you do visit a therapist, make sure—preferably by phone *before* the first session—that the therapist understands chronic illness and regularly treats people with chronic medical conditions. If you can find someone with a CFS or FM specialization, that's even better, but don't count on it. Provide your therapist with educational materials about your illness. You can even develop a treatment plan with the therapist using the techniques contained in this book. (A cognitive behavioral orientation is most compatible with the types of recommendations I offer.)

Positive Change Is Possible

Regardless of your level of functioning, you can individualize the seven steps so that they fit into your lifestyle. Of course, any positive change you make will probably require a rethinking of how you do your daily activities. Rethinking is good—rethinking leads to open-mindedness and flexibility, which will allow you to experiment with your daily schedule and produce a better balance among activity, rest, and leisure. This is where you want to be.

CHAPTER 15

Test Yourself: The Improvement Checklist

The checklist below targets key elements of your thinking and lifestyle that are related to improving or worsening illness. Assess your agreement with the following statements; respond to each item with a yes or no. (I will review each of the thirteen items directly after the checklist.)

1. I overdo my activities relative to my energy level.

2. I pace my activities—that is, I do tasks in small chunks rather than doing them all at once.

3. I do much more when I feel better and much less when I feel worse.

4. I keep regular hours for going to bed at night and getting up in the morning.

5. I must get well in order to experience a good quality of life.

6. I often feel angry, frustrated, or depressed about being ill.

7. I feel a lot of guilt over what I cannot do.

8. Being viewed by other people as a nice or good person is essential to me.

9. Quiet relaxation is an important activity in my life.

10. I can usually express my negative feelings to others.

11. I have many pleasant experiences in my life.

12. I have many more negative experiences than positive experiences.

13. I receive good emotional support from others.

1. I overdo my activities relative to my energy level.

Overdoing activities seems to be almost universal in people with CFS and FM. (Even if you are quite limited, you can still overdo activities relative to the energy you have.) You probably would have strongly agreed with this statement when you were well; now, you may be doing a lot less, but may still be exhausting yourself. If you disagree with this item, then you may have finally put the brakes on the do-it-all, finish-it-all attitude—this, of course, is where you want to be!

2. I pace my activities—that is, I do tasks in small chunks rather than doing them all at once.

In a sense, this is the opposite of the previous statement. The more you agree with this statement, the better; this means that instead of overdoing and exhausting yourself, you're pacing your activities, thus maintaining—or even slowly increasing—your energy levels.

3. I do much more when I feel better and much less when I feel worse.

This is the classic up-and-down, push-crash pattern, an understandable but vicious cycle that only perpetuates frustration. The less you agree with this statement the better. A better goal: avoid the ups and downs by keeping to your usual activities. Don't do a lot more on a good day or a lot less on a bad day.

4. I keep regular hours for going to bed at night and getting up in the morning.

You want to be in agreement with this statement. Treatment studies of sleep disorders show that regular bedtime hours with a minimum of daytime napping is conducive to more restful sleep. (Not necessarily totally refreshing sleep, but at least better sleep.) No matter how sick you may be, the practice of good sleep techniques (see chapter 8) is crucial to recovering energy.

5. I must get well in order to experience a good quality of life.

This attitude is the bugaboo of many people with CFS and FM. You don't want to agree with this statement. Why? Because the demand to get well can lead to desperate measures—anything from an endless hunt for remedies and cures to a blanket denial of illness, propped up by caffeine, forced activity, and energy-draining attempts to ignore symptoms. A better attitude would be: "I would like to be well, but short of that, I can still design my life to be as satisfying as possible."

6. I often feel angry, frustrated, or depressed about being ill.

These are understandable emotions when you have a chronic illness; in no way do I intend to downplay the feelings of devastation you may have. However, these emotions reflect a deep intolerance of ongoing symptoms. Yes, it's unfair—in fact, it's a particularly cruel irony given the high energy and productivity levels you used to have. But it's also an unfortunate reality. The less you agree with this statement the better.

7. I feel a lot of guilt over what I cannot do.

Again, this is an understandable reaction to your limitations. However, you can choose to focus on what you can still do—however little that may be—instead. That's all you can reasonably ask of yourself. The less guilt the better. The less you agree with this statement the better.

8. Being viewed by other people as a nice or good person is essential to me.

People with CFS and FM often want to be viewed as nice or good people. It's when you absolutely *must* be viewed this way that stress is generated. If you let being viewed as nice become more important to you than taking care of yourself, you drain your energy even more. Putting limits on our "goodism" helps to preserve ourselves. What do you lose? Perhaps other people won't think you're nice all of the time. Is that devastating? I don't think so. Besides, having everyone at all times thinking you're nice is an unrealistic goal anyway. The less you agree with this statement the better.

9. Quiet relaxation is an important activity in my life.

Devoting a good period of time daily to relaxation is important to your health and well-being. The more you can honestly agree with this statement the better.

10. I can usually express my negative feelings to others.

For many people with CFS or FM, this doesn't come naturally. What usually happens is that negative feelings are held back for fear of alienating someone or causing conflict. However, the negative feelings that you suppress linger on inside you and create stress—studies have shown that abnormalities in stress hormone levels in people with CFS and FM may be related to pent-up negative feelings. When you express your negative feelings you release your stress. That is positive and healthy. The more you agree with this statement the better.

11. I have many pleasant experiences in my life.

Pleasant experiences lead to improvements; and pleasant experiences that require less exertion are even better. Pleasant events can counteract distress and ongoing symptoms by producing feelings of joy, wonder, enthusiasm—all of which not only distract from symptoms, but can even lessen their severity. You definitely want to be in agreement with this statement.

12. I have many more negative experiences than positive experiences.

If this statement is true for you, then you need to shift your activities until your positive experiences outweigh your negative ones. Positive experiences are important in and of themselves, but if they're outweighed by negative ones, any potential benefits may be significantly reduced. You want to be in disagreement with this statement.

13. I receive good emotional support from others.

If you don't have sensitive, understanding others around you, you may receive too little support. On the other hand, if you find yourself talking to sympathetic others about your illness all the time, you may be receiving too much support. (Too much support can make you feel like an invalid who can only do very little.) A good level of support is enough to feel connected, but not so much that you feel disabled. You want to be in agreement with this statement.

The thirteen items on this checklist represent the key factors related to improving (or worsening) your illness. I recommend that you prioritize these items; work on only a few at a time—don't let yourself get overwhelmed by tackling all thirteen at once. Here are some suggestions for weekly assignments (based on the seven steps) to help you get started:

Weeks 1 and 2: Begin regular relaxation practice.

Weeks 3 and 4: Introduce pacing into your daily schedule.

Weeks 5 and 6: Design a healthy sleep routine; implement it on a daily basis.

Weeks 7 and 8: Practice expressing negative feelings to others when they arise. (These could include requests for more support and refusals to do things that overtax you.)

Weeks 9 and 10: Practice coping statements; allow yourself to realize that you don't have to be all things to all people.

Weeks 11 and 12: Make a list of low-effort pleasant activities to do; schedule them for several times a week—and eventually for several times a day.

Weeks 13 and 14: Use coping statements to let go of any insistence that you must get well in order to have a good quality of life; take charge of your own personal improvement effort.

CHAPTER 16

How to Make Yourself Miserable

The title of this chapter was taken from an old comedy book by Dan Greenberg, a humorous counterpoint to self-help books that emphasized positive thinking—after all, if you can learn to think straight, you should also be able to learn to think crooked! I know it's not always easy to see the lighter side of these illnesses, but remember: your reactions to your illness are based on the decisions *you* make, conscious or unconscious, about how the illness fits into your life.

Having CFS or FM can certainly be an unpleasant, life-altering event, but to truly be miserable, you have to think the right thoughts, too.

Nine Rules to Ensure CFS/FM Misery

1. Ask yourself, "Why me?" as often as possible. Whenever you feel any degree of peace, know that this is a false

peace—you are still ill; you must endlessly question why this curse has been visited upon you.

2. Focus on how sick you are; magnify every ache, pain, flu-like feeling, or discomfort that you have—to the greatest degree possible. Only in this way will you realize the true impact of your illness.

3. As an alternative approach, ignore—and deny—all of your symptoms. Consume as much caffeine as necessary to power you through the day. After all, ignoring your illness is the only way to feel normal and healthy!

4. View relapses and setbacks as your body betraying you; this illness obviously has nothing to do with you or your lifestyle. View it as a foreign invasion—as if aliens have just taken over your body.

5. Look to physicians, medical researchers, and other healers for your salvation. After all, only they can improve your life, and only they can possibly have a clue about how to lessen your symptoms. Reject any personal efforts to change your life as simply cosmetic. Remember: a complete cure is the only acceptable outcome.

6. Be as mad at yourself as you possibly can be for not being able to make yourself well. Also, be mad at anyone and everyone who doesn't understand your illness—what's there not to understand in an illness that's invisible, not recognized by doctors, and has no identified cause or effective treatment?

7. Declare yourself inadequate because you cannot do things or help others the way you used to. After all, if you cannot meet your own high standards now that you're ill, you must be even more inadequate than when you were well and doing more.

8. View relaxing thoughts as satanic—banish them immediately from your consciousness. Replace them with thoughts of all the things that you'd like to do but know that you can't do. Keep your mind focused firmly on the happy days of the past, when you were well. Remember

those days as blissful and carefree yet highly productive. Never question your old priorities—they were indisputably the correct ones.

9. View guilt, anxiety, and frustration as your dearest friends that prove how intolerable life is with your illness.

Okay, I doubt that anyone really buys into *all* of these purposely exaggerated beliefs. But you may buy into some of them, at least at some level. I know I firmly believed points 4 and 5 until a few years ago: I viewed setbacks with loathing and intolerance and looked to any number of medical and alternative treatments to cure me; nothing less was acceptable.

Don't Overinvest Negative Emotions in These Illnesses

For those of you who think I'm demeaning the legitimacy of CFS and FM, let me assure you that I would never dismiss the major impact of these illnesses on people's lives. I myself have CFS; I truly do understand the impact it has. On the other hand, the more negative emotion and thought that you invest in your illness, the more it will dominate your life.

A very good quality of life is still possible, even with these illnesses—and a good quality of life can, in turn, lead to illness improvement. This is the track that you want to be on. So, if I spoof those of us who get mired in illness turmoil sometimes, it's only to coax you to step back from your illness and recognize the part that you, yourself, are playing in equating fatigue and pain with suffering. One does not have to equal the other.

The irony is that when you stop fighting and struggling against these illnesses, your chances for improvement increase. I know this from firsthand experience: for more than a decade I made myself miserable with some of the above beliefs. I rarely do that anymore. The result: I feel much less frustration, my illness has diminished, and my quality of life has improved—a lot. This is where you want to be, too.

PART III

Physicians, Treatments, and "Cures"

This final section highlights several important issues. For one thing, the relationship you have with your physician can affect both how you feel about your illness and the progress you make toward improvement (chapter 17). Your illness will also be influenced—for better or worse—by the treatments you try, whether they be medical, alternative, or behavioral (chapters 18 and 19). And ultimately, your attitudes about cures and healing will have a powerful impact on your quality of life (chapter 20).

CHAPTER 17

Physician Visits: Why They Go Wrong

One of the most troubling aspects of having CFS and FM is a difficulty in finding a knowledgeable, sensitive physician to diagnose and treat the condition. The skepticism, condescension, and even ridicule of some doctors can be as devastating as the illnesses themselves. And yet, most patients want a medical diagnosis: a diagnosis of CFS or FM can both validate perplexing symptoms and reassure you that the illness is not life-threatening.

However, problems abound with physician visits. First of all, physicians who don't believe in these illnesses may refuse to provide treatment or ongoing care. (This makes sense: if you don't believe in an illness, how can you treat the patient?) Secondly, physicians may not offer any real help simply because they don't know what to do. (Being told that you are just depressed is usually not a cause for joy and cathartic renewal.)

Physicians, as a whole, are generally more comfortable with medical problems that reveal themselves in laboratory tests and respond to conventional treatments. This is, in part, because physicians view illness in the same mind-body terms that people with CFS and FM do—physicians are just as beholden to their diagnostic tests as the rest of us, believing that only these tests will "prove" that we are ill.

Physicians and the Psychiatric Model

Many articles have been published in the medical literature by physicians who view CFS and FM as psychiatric conditions. I wouldn't deny that there are psychiatric aspects to our illnesses; however, the reduction of these illnesses to psychiatric disorders reflects the outdated medical view that illnesses are of either the mind or the body—an integrated mind-body model is simply rejected. However, for the major diseases of our time—including heart disease, cancer, and diabetes—evidence shows that psychological and lifestyle factors play important roles.

In 1999, Arthur Barsky and Jonathan Borus, both psychiatrists at Harvard Medical School, published a lightning-rod article titled "Functional Somatic Syndromes" in the *Annals of Internal Medicine*. In it, they grouped CFS, FM, multiple chemical sensitivities, irritable bowel syndrome, and several other illnesses together as *functional somatic syndromes* (illnesses that cannot be explained by known medical conditions). They argued that the symptoms of these illnesses are maintained solely by the belief that one has a serious disease; that this belief itself causes patients to dwell on symptoms and amplify them to alarming levels.

I don't dispute that certain beliefs and emotions do play a role in the symptoms that you experience. This is not a denial of the reality of these illnesses—beliefs influence how you react to any medical condition, from heart disease to cancer.

What Doctors Recommend to Other Doctors About CFS/FM

Barsky and Borus advise practicing physicians to do standard medical workups on these patients and then search for diagnosable psychiatric disorders (standard protocol in medical evaluations). The authors then suggest therapeutic lines of communication between physician and patient, emphasizing sensitivity to the patient's suffering. The irony here is that these skeptical physicians actually advocate the type of care that you would want to receive from physicians! This is what they specifically recommend to doctors treating patients with illnesses such as CFS and FM:

> ... a collaborative therapeutic alliance between physician and patient is crucial. The physician must take special care to acknowledge and legitimize the patient's suffering because a definitive biomedical explanation for the patient's symptoms has proven elusive. At the same time, the physician should discourage the patient from assuming a passive role, should undercut false expectations about the clinical course, and should avoid making distressing symptom attributions. Closely related to the establishment of collaborative alliance is the process of making symptom palliation, coping and reha-bilitation the focus of the clinical enterprise. If this is to be accomplished, patients with functional somatic syndromes must be actively involved in the treatment process and must be dissuaded from assuming a passive role in waiting to be cured by medical procedures or interventions (917).

It doesn't sound that unreasonable, does it? You may object to some parts of what they've said, but overall, the approach advocated here is to work with the patient. These authors deserve credit for attempting to legitimize the patient's presentation rather than simply dismissing it. Yet how many of you have ever encountered a physician who is willing to take this approach? Unfortunately, despite all of this high-minded talk about *working with* these patients, few physicians actually do this. In fact, the personal reports that I've received—as well as published studies—indicate quite the opposite. Such a constructive approach to helping the patient is sadly absent.

Your Right to Be Skeptical

The problem with physicians was well-stated by a thirty-five-year-old attorney with CFS:

The bottom line is that physicians, in general, don't want to spend their time with us because of the difficulties in diagnosis, treatment, and ongoing care. Let's be honest and just acknowledge this rather than hide behind ivory tower pronouncements of feigned concern. The Hippocratic oath, which many physicians take on entering their profession, states, "First, do no harm . . ." We don't ask for a cure, we know it's not out there yet—but don't worsen our burdens with your attitudes of arrogance. If you don't know how to treat us, say so rather than taking the easy way out by affixing a one-size-fits-all psychiatric label and then referring us to a mental health professional who hasn't a clue how to treat these conditions. If you want to refer us to a specialist, including a mental health specialist, make sure it's someone who has an interest in and understanding of these conditions.

The Role of Doctors in Discouraging Healing Possibilities

Because doctors often categorize CFS and FM as psychiatric disorders or non-illnesses, they often fail to offer any kind of plan of action that might be helpful. Instead, they may fall back on useless medical clichés, in effect, dismissing your concerns. The outcome of your medical visit may thus be a referral to a mental health professional or empty reassurance that nothing is wrong. Given physicians' skeptical attitudes, it's hardly surprising that many patients come to view mental health treatment and behavioral change as quasi-treatments for malingerers and complainers. As a result, people with CFS and FM may become ever more desperate for medical validation and effective treatment.

The Modern Medical Myth: Most Illnesses Have Identified Causes

Although physicians seek to identify illnesses with a variety of diagnostic tests, they often don't succeed. For instance, it's estimated that up to 85 percent of patients with lower back pain have no definitive diagnosis (Long et al. 1996). In fact, a large percentage of patients who visit physicians are deemed as not having medically understood conditions. Should all of these patients then be referred to psychiatrists or other mental health professionals? Would that really be helpful?

Many psychiatrists—and other mental health professionals, too—also view CFS (and to a lesser extent FM) as a non-illness. Thus, patients are often dropped or referred to other practitioners who may or may not be able to help. I don't blame individual physicians; this behavior simply reflects their medical school training—as well, perhaps, as the god-like omniscience that many patients demand of them. But physicians don't have all the answers.

The Physician's View

Let me take the side of the physicians for a moment: you present your complaints to them—complaints which elude definitive diagnosis or effective treatment. What are they to do? Yes, there are symptom-managing medications that may be helpful for some, but for many this treatment is ineffective. It's a lose-lose proposition for a physician. For any treatment they offer, improvement will probably be slight at best. On the other hand, if they choose not to treat, they may feel they have failed. And if you convey the attitude that only a physician can help you, the pressure the physician feels may only increase.

The CFIDS Association of America has undertaken a highly laudable effort to educate physicians about diagnosis and treatment of CFS (this effort is currently ongoing); perhaps in time this will help to improve communication between CFS/FM patients and their doctors. For now, it still remains largely in *your* hands to take control of your illness as much as you can.

Physician Skepticism: Does the Diagnosis Perpetuate the Condition?

Many physicians fear that diagnosing CFS or FM will actually help perpetuate these illnesses. We might call Edward Shorter, a physician who writes about psychosomatic conditions, the dean of this anti-diagnosis school:

> Virtually all [CFS patients are] medically well individuals in the grips of the delusion that they [are ill]. Supposed new

diseases such as CFS flourish in the subcultures of hypochondriasis that form within patient support groups. The caregivers themselves contribute to their patients' somatic fixations, plunging youthful and productive people into careers of disability. In every large community there will be found at least one physician willing to play up to his patients' psychological need for organicity. The mainline press has picked up [and often endorsed] these goofy illness attributions (1995, 116–118).

There is at least one study in CFS which confirms that this negative viewpoint is common (Woodward, Broom, and Legge 1995). Seventeen out of twenty physicians interviewed in this study believed that a diagnosis of CFS or FM would become a self-fulfilling prophecy of continued symptoms and disability for those so diagnosed. Similarly, during an MSNBC program about FM (2000), neurologist Thomas Bohr stated that a diagnosis of FM convinces patients that they are invalids. He then asked a conference room full of his fellow neurologists how many of them thought that FM was *not* a useful diagnosis—almost the entire room raised their hands in agreement as chuckles pervaded the room.

Arguments For and Against Withholding Diagnosis

The main argument for withholding a diagnosis for these illnesses is that the diagnosis itself may be an important factor in perpetuating disability. However, it's difficult to determine if disability has, indeed, been perpetuated by the diagnosis itself unless the diagnosis can somehow be taken back. In a way, this is what was done in a cognitive behavioral treatment study of people with CFS conducted by Michael Sharpe and his colleagues (1996). In this study, part of the treatment patients received was to convince them that they weren't actually suffering from any organic disease. (This should sound familiar.) The goal was to focus patients on self-control of symptoms, rather than reliance on doctors. The treatment was quite successful and the patients reported significant reductions in symptoms and improvements in functioning. Was the effort to persuade patients that they did not have a disease the reason why they improved?

This question was answered, in part, by a later, similar cognitive behavioral treatment study conducted by Alicia Deale and her colleagues (1997). In their approach to treatment, they made *no* attempt to persuade patients that they did not have a disease. Yet, the CFS patients in the Deale study actually showed *greater* improvements than those in the Sharpe study. Clearly, attempting to convince patients they aren't medically ill isn't essential for people to benefit from treatment. So doctors who attempt to convince you that you're not ill probably aren't being helpful—if anything, such pronouncements will probably just make you more determined to find out what you have and what you can do about it.

Also, people with CFS and FM may endure years of debilitating symptoms before they are diagnosed. If the formal diagnosis itself is what perpetuates the illness, how is it that individuals may suffer unremitting symptoms for years *prior* to diagnosis? In the last five years, I've been contacted by many people suffering from CFS—people who only became aware of their formal diagnosis through participation in my research. Although they had been ill for years, they didn't have any idea that CFS applied to them; clearly, the absence of a diagnosis hadn't prevented them from becoming persistently ill.

Do Symptoms and Impairments Change After a Diagnosis?

One recent Canadian study did explore how symptoms and disabilities change after a diagnosis of FM is made. In this study, Kevin White and his colleagues (2002) evaluated fifty-six patients newly diagnosed with FM. These same patients were then reevaluated eighteen to thirty-six months later. At these follow-up evaluations, no changes were found in physical function or health care utilization. In addition, these patients actually reported *fewer* symptoms as well as a significant improvement in health satisfaction. So these individuals, after receiving the diagnosis of FM, not only did no worse, they actually seemed to do somewhat better! This is the first study (at least, that I'm aware of) that directly tested the hypothesis that a diagnosis of CFS or FM perpetuates these conditions; its findings decidedly do not support the antidiagnosis argument. If this type of study is replicated— perhaps with a "no diagnosis" control condition—physicians may, at long last, take notice.

Finally, I have found no study that shows that withholding a diagnosis and referring patients to mental health professionals actually helps people with these illnesses; although skeptical physicians may refuse to diagnose CFS and FM, many of them do not offer any alternatives for dealing with these illnesses.

How Doctors Can Help

So how, then, should physicians medically treat people with CFS and FM? We don't have a good answer to this yet, although the prescription of medications for some level of symptom relief would seem to constitute a useful approach, at least in part. In the meantime, my colleagues, Leonard Jason and Charles Lapp, are teaching physicians across the country how to properly diagnose CFS and establish therapeutic alliances with patients.

Establishing a therapeutic alliance between physicians and patients is a basic but necessary step. In an article published in the *British Journal of General Practice* (1999), Heather Elliot grappled with how physicians should best approach patients with these illnesses. She suggested that although people with CFS (and FM) may be resistant to psychological diagnoses, they may still be willing to acknowledge a role for stress in their illnesses. Thus, physicians could support the legitimacy of CFS and FM while at the same time identifying stress factors.

Sometimes, an alliance between physician and patient can be enough in and of itself to lead to improvement. A study by Barbara Saltzstein and her colleagues (1998) found that women with CFS who were believed and supported by their physicians tended to have better outcomes over the long term; even in the absence of a specific treatment, a physician's positive prognosis was related to the patient's having hope—and, ultimately, showing improvement or recovery. This is not to say that a good relationship with your doctor is a cure for CFS or FM, but rather that through social connection and support your doctor can provide some level of optimism, understanding, and direction for you.

Combining Medical and Behavioral Approaches

As I have emphasized, behavioral assessment is very important in identifying the lifestyle factors that may help to sustain your illness.

However, most physicians aren't trained in behavioral assessment—nor do they have the time to make a meticulous analysis of a patient's lifestyle.

Ideally, physicians and psychologists would work with patients together, thus addressing both the medical and the behavioral aspects of these illnesses simultaneously—and thus greatly enhancing the chances for improvement. Physicians Peter Madill and David Klonoff are attempting such an endeavor, using a combination of medical and group support techniques with their CFS patients; so far, they've reported encouraging findings at several chronic fatigue conferences.

Your question at this point may be: where do I find such a doctor? My recommendation is that you contact your local CFS/FM support organization—they should have an appropriate referral list for your area.

CHAPTER 18

Medical and Alternative Treatments

No medical treatments have been developed specifically for CFS or FM. Drug treatments by themselves may benefit only a minority of patients; and unfortunately, drug hypersensitivity and adverse reactions to medications are not uncommon. Cognitive behavioral treatments may well benefit people with CFS and FM, but still, even for those who experience improvement, recovery is rare.

Medical Treatments for CFS

In the absence of a cure for CFS, studies have explored treatment of its symptoms. Ampligen, an immune-boosting drug, has shown promise in one such controlled study (Strayer et al. 1994). On the other hand, a survey of Ampligen patients in the *National Forum* (Kansky and Tai 1999) revealed poor outcomes and adverse reactions in many patients. Clearly, Ampligen needs further study.

Because fatigue and depression are often linked, physicians sometimes prescribe antidepressants for CFS patients. However, two controlled studies of Prozac in CFS patients have reported no beneficial effect on CFS or depression symptoms (Wearden et al. 1998; Vercoulen, Swanink, Zitman, et al. 1996). This doesn't mean that antidepressants aren't helpful for some people with CFS. In fact, a survey I did of 285 CFS patients (Friedberg 1995) revealed that roughly one in four respondents did indeed report significant benefits from antidepressant medications. On the other hand, 31 percent of respondents said that antidepressants made them feel worse.

In a different approach to treating CFS, some physicians have found that people with CFS frequently have low blood pressure. Following up on this possible link, a diagnostic test known as the *tilt table test* has shown that a small percentage of people with CFS also have a blood pressure abnormality called *neurally mediated hypotension*. Although an early study of medication treatment for this blood pressure abnormality was encouraging, it's not clear how effective this treatment is; moreover, many physicians who treat CFS haven't found this blood pressure problem in their patients.

Alternative Treatments for CFS

Initial studies of some alternative therapies for CFS have shown promise as symptom-reduction treatments. Perhaps the most impressive to date is massage. In a well-designed study of massage therapy and CFS conducted by Tiffany Field and colleagues (1997), people who received massage reported significant reductions in fatigue, pain, and stress—and had improved sleep as well. Of course, massage is expensive and rarely covered by health insurance; however, the patients I know who get regular massages report very substantial benefits. In addition to the physical effects of the massage itself, taking that time for yourself is also healthy and stress-reducing in and of itself. (This is consistent with the seven-step approach.)

Another potentially promising alternative treatment is essential fatty acids, such as primrose oil. Two controlled studies of essential fatty acids and CFS have found significant improvement in illness conditions (Behan, Behan, and Horrobin 1990; Plioplys and Plioplys 1997), although a later controlled study (Warren, McKendrick, and

Peet 1999) failed to replicate these earlier findings; this supplement requires further testing and study.

Any number of other alternative treatments are also available for people with CFS and other poorly understood chronic conditions, including homeopathy, shark cartilage supplements, blue-green algae supplements, vitamin/mineral/amino acid supplements, magnet therapy, and clinical ecology. However, none of these alternative treatments has been evaluated in published studies.

In my previous book on CFS, *Coping With Chronic Fatigue Syndrome: Nine Things You Can Do* (1995), I had patients rate a number of these treatments. Antiallergy and antiyeast diets, biofeedback, and stress management were among the most helpful treatments, with 24 to 30 percent giving these approaches ratings of favorable to highly favorable.

Concerns About Alternative Treatments

Please understand that alternative treatments aren't necessarily harmless. Even herbs and vitamins can cause side effects and adverse reactions in certain individuals. Personally, I'm leery of claims that an herb must be harmless just because it has been used in another culture for thousands of years. Herbs are multi-ingredient compounds that, for the most part, haven't been scientifically tested. In general, I'm skeptical of any new, unproven treatment for two reasons: first, many people with CFS and FM have been hurt by unproven treatments; second, patients often spend a lot of money on treatments that produce temporary improvements at best. This is not to dissuade you from trying any type of therapy, drug, supplement, or other approach that you think may work. My voiced concerns are only intended as a cautious advisory to those who are considering new treatments.

Another element to bear in mind is the placebo effect. This may occur with whatever treatment you try, whether it has been previously tested or not. The placebo effect may cause you to feel better temporarily, simply as a result of your own expectations and beliefs that you'll feel better. When drug treatment trials are run with placebo controls, the placebo effect is often found to be almost as powerful as the drug itself. This is why it's so important to have a placebo control condition; a treatment can be deemed effective only if it is significantly better than the placebo alone. Apart from placebo effects, it can be difficult to differentiate real treatment effects from the occasional improvements in your illness condition that can occur naturally anyway, without treatment.

Medical Treatments for FM

Published reviews of treatment studies in FM suggest that both drug and nondrug treatments can be helpful to some degree. Yet in real terms, only about 40 percent of people with FM benefit from these treatments. (Yes, that's still a lot better than zero!)

In contrast to antidepressant studies in CFS, antidepressant medication and muscle relaxants *do* reduce symptoms and emotional stress in some people with FM. On the other hand, nonsteroidal, anti-inflammatory drugs—e.g., ibuprofen—*haven't* been effective in treating these types of symptoms. Also, antidepressants that increase serotonin levels (e.g., tricyclic Elavil) may improve sleep and reduce pain in FM.

A study by Donald Goldenberg—a renowned FM expert at the Newton-Wellesley Hospital in Boston—and his colleagues (1996) found that a combination of two antidepressants, amitriptyline (Elavil) and fluoxetine (Prozac), significantly reduced pain, improved sleep, and increased well-being in FM patients; the combination of the two drugs worked significantly better than either did alone.

Physicians prescribing drug treatments for patients with FM must be willing to adjust dosages and try different medications in different combinations to identify the most effective approach for each patient.

Alternative Treatments for FM

Because you may be one of the 60 percent of FM patients for whom medical therapies don't work, you may find it worthwhile to look into alternative treatments. At least one alternative pain-reduction therapy seems to show promise: SAMe (S-adenosyl-L-methionine), an over-the-counter supplement, has been found to reduce depression, pain, and the number of tender points in FM patients in two controlled studies (Jacobsen et al. 1991; Volkmann et al. 1997). On the other hand, a controlled study of the alternative treatment Super Malic—a combination of malic acid and magnesium—found no positive benefits in people with FM (Russell et al. 1995). In addition, a recent well-controlled study of acupuncture in fibromyalgia (Assefi et al. 2005) found that the technique was no more effective than a sham accupuncture treatment.

Two other alternative treatments may also have benefits for FM patients. A six-month study of a warm-water pool exercise program for people with FM (Mannerkorpi et al. 2000) found significant reductions in FM symptoms, improved physical endurance, lessened pain severity and stress, and improved quality of life—both at the end of treatment and at a follow-up assessment two years later. These findings make sense: doing gentle stretching and relaxation exercises in a warm pool can be a wonderfully soothing activity. However, this is probably something you need to do regularly to maintain benefits.

CHAPTER 19

Graded Activity and Exercise: Improved Coping or Improved Illness?

The aim of graded activity treatment—a type of cognitive behavioral therapy—is to help individuals with CFS and FM overcome any reluctance to becoming more active, and then gradually increase activity levels. Graded activity and graded exercise are somewhat controversial, because these techniques seem to suggest that people can be cured of these illnesses solely by psychological treatment. Understandably, patient advocacy organizations have protested that graded activity alone cannot cure these illnesses. Some activists also fear that the successes of graded activity treatment might be used as evidence that these illnesses are psychiatric disorders, thus discouraging further research on illness causes and medical treatment.

As of yet, there hasn't been a well-designed study of graded activity done in the U.S., although several have been conducted in Europe (more below). Leonard Jason, a well-known CFS expert, is currently conducting such a study at DePaul University in Chicago. (The study is actually a head-to-head comparison of all of the major forms of lifestyle treatment for CFS; in addition to a graded activity condition, three other treatments are also being tested in this study: a coping skills condition, a stretching exercise condition, and an active relaxation treatment. Results won't be available until late 2006.)

I believe that graded activity can be helpful for some people with CFS and FM; graded activity can be quite successfully integrated with the pacing techniques described in chapter 9. Initially, only very small amounts of activity—such as five to ten minutes of walking a day—are prescribed. (This is consistent with breaking tasks into small steps, a key characteristic of pacing.) As tolerance develops, higher activity prescriptions can then be assigned.

One reason why graded activity may work is because it represents time taken for one's self—an important aspect of the seven-step approach.

The European Graded Activity Treatment Studies

Between 1996 and 2001, three well-designed studies (Deale et al 1997; Prins et al. 2001; Sharpe et al. 1996) of graded activity treatment in CFS were published in Europe. These studies made use of other cognitive and behavioral techniques as well, such as sleep improvement strategies and cognitive therapy to reduce excessive perfectionism and stressful thinking. On the face of it, it doesn't seem as if such simple treatment could possibly be effective in a condition as severe as CFS. Yet there were improvements—big improvements—in functioning for the majority of patients in these studies, as well as substantial reductions in fatigue.

This suggests that some percentage of patients did, indeed, respond positively to increasing their overall level of activity—in part, presumably, because they were helped to overcome unrealistic fears of symptom flare-ups. However, by and large, these studies didn't treat higher-functioning, working individuals. The great majority of the patients in these studies were unable to work; many of these individuals were less active than they needed to be. Most people with CFS in the U.S., however, are in the higher-functioning category, and it's not clear whether simply increasing your physical activity when you're already active will lead to improvement. Yet in the pilot work I'm now doing, even high functioning individuals with CFS seem to benefit from low level daily walking.

Why Personal Graded Activity Programs May Fail

In your own personal efforts to be more active, you may fail to truly pace yourself; even without meaning to, you may do a lot more when you feel better and a lot less when you feel worse. By comparison, all of the graded activity treatment studies built a very strict pacing of activities into their treatment plans—in fact, for some individuals, daily activity was actually *reduced* at the start of treatment because they were doing too much.

It's very difficult to both keep to a strict schedule of pacing and, at the same time, slowly increase activity over several months, all on your own. When I told one of my CFS patients, a thirty-seven-year-old screenwriter on disability, to increase his walking time by five minutes a week, he responded, "Five minutes a week! Are you kidding? I want to build myself up, but this will take forever. I have to get back to work or just be more active—this is just going to take too long."

Exercise as Therapy: Can It Work?

Although low-level graded activity may seem, in principle, like a reasonable way of building yourself up when you're ill with CFS, if exercise was your passion when you were well, low-level graded activity may pale in comparison. At this point, you're probably very familiar with the endless frustration of not being able to do your exercise; even if you can still exercise in some limited way, there's almost certainly an upper limit on how much you can do, and the energy and good feelings that used to come from aerobic workouts are probably much less than they used to be. Before we return to graded activity, let's discuss this exercise issue—first, with an example of too much aerobic exercise, and then with a potentially useful alternative: anaerobic exercise.

■ Cindy's Story: The Consequences of Too Much Exercise, Too Soon

Cindy, a twenty-eight-year-old colleague of mine, thought she was recovered from a five-year bout with CFS. Very excited, she made the mistake of ignoring the limits of what she could do: she celebrated her recovery by resuming the four miles of powerwalking she used to do every day. For thirty days, she powerwalked—and then relapsed into illness. This was a huge blow to her, particularly after feeling so well.

It's easy to understand why Cindy immediately jumped back into her old pre-CFS exercise routine. The pent-up desire to do things can be very strong—it can be a real challenge to limit yourself and do less when you feel that you can do much more. But you may never again be your old, high energy self. Gradualism and pacing should guide your activity; anticipate falling down *before* it happens, don't just push ahead and hope that it doesn't happen.

Because standard (nongraded) aerobic exercise—such as walking or jogging—may be difficult to tolerate, one possible solution may be to focus on *anaerobic* exercise—such as stretching or mild weight-lifting— instead. Anaerobic exercise aims to increase strength and improve flexibility. Low-level anaerobic exercise can relax you and may increase your energy; it may also have the added benefit of both reducing muscle pain and increasing a sense of well-being. However, please, please do not make it your goal to do a high level of nonaerobic exercise every day to somehow substitute for other exercise that you can't do! When you pressure yourself, you risk losing any progress you've already made.

To make an anaerobic exercise program work, you must start at a very low level and only very slowly increase the exercise intensity, allowing yourself adequate time for recovery between sessions. Arnold Van Ness, an exercise physiologist and CFS expert, suggests practicing a series of *range of motion exercises*, such as hamstring stretches, lateral bends, and lower back stretches; these types of exercises can improve flexibility, decrease joint pain, and enhance overall functioning. More-over, *light resistance exercises*, such as modified push-ups, sit-ups, and flex-knee crunches, can also help build and maintain strength. Van Ness suggests very brief periods of exercise—thirty seconds or less—followed by at least one minute of rest (or until full muscle recovery is achieved); a single session shouldn't exceed twenty minutes.

Does Graded Activity Increase Activity or Just Rearrange It?

Although patients in the graded activity studies were told to gradually do more, it's not clear if that's what actually happened. In two of the studies, activity levels weren't measured objectively. In the third study, in which activity levels *were* objectively measured, no change was found in overall activity levels after treatment; the assumption that people are doing more after treatment simply wasn't confirmed.

Over the past year, I've used activity monitors in twelve people with CFS and FM to further test this assumption. These individuals were treated with a combination of the seven-step program and graded activity. After, on average, only seven-and-a-half hours of this intervention, six out of the eight reported improvement. However, the activity monitor data revealed no significant increase in physical activity—in fact, according to the data, activity levels actually decreased slightly.

Why, then, were the subjects saying they had improved? The next section may provide at least part of the answer.

▪ Richard's Story: A Test of Graded Activity Treatment

Richard, a fifty-two-year-old CFS patient, allowed me to collect data on him to discover if he actually increased his activity level during a graded activity treatment program (Friedberg 2002). Richard was able to work full-time, but had given up all physical exercise because of symptom flare-ups. His graded activity schedule began with a five-minute walk every other day; over a one-year period, we increased this to a thirty-minute walk every day. (Do you get the idea of what *gradual* means in this context now?) He was able to follow this schedule without flare-ups—a major improvement in and of itself.

To measure his physical activity levels throughout the treatment, Richard wore a pedometer. At the start of his treatment, Richard did *no* regular walking. By the end of the treatment he was walking for thirty minutes every day. It would seem that Richard's activity level had increased quite substantially. However, surprisingly, his step counts at the end of treatment were actually 10 percent *less* than they were at the beginning of treatment. At the same time, it seemed as if the treatment really was working: Richard rated himself as "much improved."

How could this be? Why would his step counts decrease when he said he was walking a lot more? And if his actual activity level was barely changed, why would he rate himself as much improved? As we discussed these issues together, I began to realize what had actually happened. Richard came into treatment at a point in his illness where he *was* able to tolerate some exercise and get the emotional boost that people normally get from it. But, as he increased his weekly exercise, something else happened that the step counter couldn't tell me: he reduced his overtime at work from fifteen hours a week to only a couple of hours a week. The overtime had been highly stressful for Richard, as well as a cause of symptom flare-ups; so, when he both reduced his overtime and increased his mood-boosting daily walks, not surprisingly, he felt a lot better, even though his actual activity level barely changed.

In this case, the graded activity treatment didn't result in an increase in overall activity. Instead, the stress-reducing activity (walking) of the graded activity treatment was substituted for a stress-increasing activity (overtime). These types of substitution—not always easy to identify or measure in research studies—may, in part, explain the successes of graded activity studies. Within the structure of graded activity treatment, people may have replaced stressful activities with positive, uplifting, and stress-reducing activities.

But I've Tried Slowly Increasing Activity— It Doesn't Work!

Many people with CFS and FM put themselves on low-level activity schedules but become frustrated when they do not improve. Now, I can't speak for everyone's illness and how it may respond to activity scheduling, but it's definitely important to troubleshoot and adjust your schedule to make sure that it is the best possible schedule for you.

■ Jim's Story: Troubleshooting an Activity Schedule

Jim, a forty-nine-year-old police officer, had had a severe case of CFS for about two-and-a-half years. His daily activity schedule included yoga-type stretching, meditative relaxation, light household chores, eating, and taking a shower. He was on disability, and although he did have the occasional doctor's appointment, otherwise he was homebound. When he first told me about his daily schedule, it struck me as reasonable and consistent, but when I asked him about the amount of time he spent doing housework or stretching, he had only a very vague idea; he didn't want to keep track of the amount of time he spent on activities because he felt it would be too much pressure.

It appeared Jim was stuck in an unhealthy up-and-down pattern, albeit a very minimal one: when Jim felt better he would try to do more—and although he didn't do a lot more, he did enough to experience a mini-crash as a result. His increased activity could be anything from ten minutes of extra stretching to forty-five minutes of additional chores.

Of course, I can understand why you want to do more when you feel better, and Jim certainly wasn't doing very much more, but still, he was stuck in an up-and-down pattern. I helped Jim divide up his activities into smaller bits he could spread throughout the day. For example, three arm stretches during a single session could instead become one stretch three times a day; forty-five minutes of housework could be divided into two or three shorter sessions.

I also suggested that Jim reduce his total amount of activity. His initial reaction to this was (not surprisingly): "What? I'm already doing almost nothing. You want me to do even less?" However, because people with CFS typically do more—sometimes a lot more—than their energy levels can tolerate, activity levels often have to be reduced at first; then, once a consistent schedule is established, slow increases can begin to be made.

The Importance of a Consistent Schedule

When I say a consistent schedule, I mean that you should be slavishly consistent in carrying out those daily activities that are at—or perhaps below—a level you believe you can do. And those activities should remain at this same level even if you feel better for a few hours or days—or even a couple of weeks. Only when your schedule has been consistent for two to four weeks should you start increasing your activity level, and then only on a very gradual basis. Without guidance, many ill individuals do not have the patience to do this. However, the graded activity concept, when properly done, can work—sometimes very effectively.

Can graded activity or gradual exercise cure CFS? No, I don't believe it can. However, for many people with CFS, these may be useful techniques that can lead to improvement.

Graded Activity Treatment Studies in FM

Two major reviews of FM treatments (Rossy et al. 1999; Sim and Adams 2002) found that nondrug therapies—including physical exercise, graded activity (or cognitive behavioral) treatments, and combinations of the two—produced significant reductions in the number of tender points, FM symptoms, and psychological distress. However, only graded activity treatments actually improved daily physical functioning; follow-up assessments found that these improvements were then successfully maintained. Graded activity treatments were actually found to be more effective in improving FM symptoms and functioning than drug treatments.

You may be skeptical about how helpful these techniques really are; you've probably already tried some type of lifestyle change or exercise and haven't seen much benefit. The reason these programs may work better than your personal efforts is because they're both highly structured and very gradual. Additionally, being in a study in and of itself builds in a certain accountability: patients in a study feel obliged to follow that study's treatment program. You may not be as committed when trying these techniques on your own.

In everyday life, it's all too easy to say you don't have the time (or the interest) to carry out such a program; if you do it at all, you may end up doing it in a start-and-stop fashion. This greatly reduces its potential benefits. Another possible explanation is that you may have mixed feelings about dedicating time to yourself for these programs; you may feel it's wrong to do these things for yourself given all the other obligations you have. Ask yourself: are you willing to devote the time to do these techniques if you know your life will improve as a result? If you feel ambivalent, your efforts will be spotty and your results not so good. If, on the other hand, you can convince yourself that self-care and self-treatment is your right, then you may begin to experience illness improvement.

In Sum: Improved Illness or Improved Coping?

When we look at all of these behavioral treatment studies, what can we conclude? Do these treatments simply lead to better coping with these illnesses—or do they actually result in improvements in the illnesses themselves?

This is a difficult question to answer since coping wasn't actually measured in any of these studies; however, in long-term studies of people with CFS and FM, those who felt more control of their illnesses improved more than those who did not feel such control (see chapter 6 for details). Since improvements in coping led directly to illness improvements, better coping versus illness improvement is probably a false dichotomy. It's more accurate to say that better coping *results* in illness improvement.

Now, you may argue that you *do* cope with your illness—but aren't seeing any improvements. This is probably true for many people with these illnesses. But ask yourself this: has your coping given you a feeling of greater control of your illness? It seems that the more control you feel, the more improvements you will see. If your coping feels merely like a weak defense against an overwhelming illness, then you're probably not feeling enough illness control to generate improvement.

Unfortunately, reports in the news media about graded activity treatment and good coping as cures are inaccurate and exaggerated: neither treatment *cures* CFS or FM. Yes, symptoms and impairments may lessen—sometimes quite substantially—but they will not disappear altogether. Also, a graded activity schedule is not the royal road to improvement in and of itself.

I think the successes of behavioral treatments are due in large part to a rebalancing of lifestyle choices, even though these therapies don't explicitly include this idea. By rebalancing, I mean finding a healthy combination of activity, rest, and leisure that lessens your symptoms. When I spoke to several of the therapy trainers from these graded activity treatment studies, they all considered balancing the lives of patients to be important for good outcomes; it seems as if much more may have been done in these studies than was reported.

If you're not caught up in the notion of cure and complete recovery, viewing these treatment studies as potentially helpful makes sense. Remember: sometimes a relatively small but healthy change can lead to a variety of other changes that together yield a more balanced, satisfying life.

CHAPTER 20

The Difference Between Healing and Cure

What end point do you envision as the ultimate goal of your illness treatment program? Your end point is probably powered by hope for a cure—but also tempered by your previous experiences with not-so-successful therapies and self-improvement efforts. What ultimate level of improvement in your illness are you willing to accept? Can you have a good quality of life if you're not cured? This final chapter examines these very important issues—issues that anyone with these illnesses must face when looking to the future.

Why We May Not Find a Simple Cure

Because CFS and FM often start with a sudden rush of flu-like symptoms, many individuals have assumed that a cure will come in the form of a drug that will eradicate these flu-like symptoms—perhaps some sort of antiviral. However, as of yet, no virus or other pathogen has been linked consistently and uniquely to either CFS or FM; no simple shot or pill remedy is available at this time.

Current evidence suggests that both CFS and FM may be related to a number of biomedical factors, including immune defects, neuroendocrine abnormalities, and sleep disturbances. Additionally, there are a number of factors that clearly aggravate these conditions, including simple physical exertion, emotional stress, demanding lifestyles, and lack of good social support. Reducing these illnesses to a single smoking gun cause is unlikely; reducing these illnesses to a single cause that will then be eradicated by a straightforward medical intervention is even more unlikely.

However, let's assume for just a moment that such a lock-and-key remedy could be found. Problems still arise: first of all, there's no telling *when* it would be found; secondly, it's extremely unlikely that a medical cure would make you invulnerable to the lifestyle factors that helped trigger your illness in the first place. Perhaps someday a genetic therapy may eliminate our susceptibility to these illnesses; right now, this is all just imagination.

Even if a major drug company decides to develop a drug treatment specifically targeted to either CFS or FM, it would still take years for a drug to advance from its initial testing stages to full FDA approval. I'm not trying to be unduly pessimistic here—this is just the unfortunate reality, and also one reason why I no longer depend on any external treatment to improve my life.

The Myth of Uninterrupted Good Health

In our culture, we've come to believe that good health isn't just desirable, it's to be expected; if we fall into a state of persistent ill health, we assume that if a cure isn't currently available, one will soon be found to restore us to total health. This unrealistic expectation probably evolved from one of the greatest successes in medical science: the conquering of infectious diseases with vaccines, immunizations, and health-restoring drugs. As a result of this great success, we've come to think of cures as naturally following a sequence of first identifying and then eliminating disease. Only when you enter the medical system with your illness do you realize how naïve this conquer-and-heal notion really is.

Dr. Lyn Payer, a noted observer of American ideas about health and illness, offered this valuable insight into how Americans view their health:

> Americans regard themselves as naturally healthy. Therefore, it stands to reason that if they become ill there must be a cause for the illness, preferably one that comes from without and can be quickly dealt with ... Such a system gives primacy to the idea that disease is some wild and hairy monster that can be locked up with diagnosis and completely ignores the European idea that the severity of the disease and consequently the need for medical intervention has also to do with [the psychological and social factors that influence the disease] (1988, 139, 143).

However, the fact of the matter is that in our culture, total health for all individuals is *not* the norm. Over sixty million people—roughly one-third of the adult population—have identifiable chronic conditions, from heart disease to cancer to diabetes to autoimmune disorders. Roughly 60 percent of people over the age of forty have a chronic condition of some kind. And these statistics don't include the people with chronic illnesses who do *not* enter the medical system. The idea of pristine health is a myth, not a norm.

Also, the belief that you can somehow maintain good health if you lead an unhealthy lifestyle is a dangerous fantasy. Oh, I'm sure there are some people with iron constitutions who may practice unhealthy behaviors and yet live long, symptom-free lives, but this is a tiny minority. Realistically, it's time to let go of all of our wishful thinking about these illnesses—namely that medical research scientists will soon have an answer, that unhealthy behavior has nothing to do with being ill, and that nothing short of complete health is acceptable to lead a high-quality life.

Why Is Recovery So Difficult?

Even if you carry out every one of the lifestyle recommendations in this book, you may still not be able to completely change your life so that everything you do is healthy.

Obligations Interfere with Recovery

One reason for this is that you have obligations to yourself and others—obligations that you may not be able to ignore, but may interfere with your quest for improvement and recovery.

In my case, I know that if I could live on a Caribbean island without responsibility, I would probably achieve a greater level of recovery. Certainly, by the end of a week-long vacation at a Caribbean resort I feel significantly better. Of course, this improvement is probably not only linked to the absence of demands and pressures, but also to healthy social contact, fun, leisure, fresh food, and clean air. (I used to think clean air and healthy food were the main reasons I felt better on vacations; now I believe these factors aren't as important as a friendly and relaxed social environment.) But again, realistically it's often impossible to spend more than a couple of weeks in such a stress-free environment.

Hypersensitivity

A second reason why recovery from these illnesses is so elusive is that the illness itself renders you highly susceptible to all forms of stress. This includes the stress of ordinary exertion, the stress of exercise, the stress of social interactions, and the stress of merely thinking or concentrating. Another way of thinking about the problem is to look at your response to physical and psychological stress: you may be hypersensitive to a broad range of things, including certain foods; pollutants in our air, water, and food; and emotional stress. Hypersensitivity means that you will overreact to many of these exposures with increased symptoms and negative emotions. And this hypersensitivity will stay with you, albeit at a lower level, even when you improve.

Thus, even though you may feel a lot better, you may still overreact to things with symptom flare-ups.

So recovery—or for that matter, improvement at any level—isn't synonymous with robust good health. It means that you can feel as good as your level of improvement allows, but you must live your life with more attention to managing your feelings and symptoms than you ever did before becoming ill.

Self-Improvement, Frustration, and Recovery

Rating your progress as too slow can be another obstacle to recovery—particularly if your frustration leads you to give up the program. But ask yourself: what's the alternative? Abandoning the program will probably cause you to fall back to where you started. So your choices are: stay on the program and devote a fair amount of time to it; or go off the program, save that time to do other things, and lose all of the progress you've already made. I sincerely wish that I had a quick and effective solution. But it just doesn't exist right now.

Recovery May Not Equal Complete Restoration of Energy

In a study of energy and fatigue in people with CFS (Wood et al. 1994), three groups were compared in terms of their energy levels: people with active CFS, people who had recovered from CFS, and normal healthy individuals. As expected, people with CFS had the lowest energy levels and the normal, healthy people had the highest. Perhaps surprisingly, the individuals who said they had recovered from CFS actually had energy levels midway between the two.

So, for those who claim to be recovered, my belief is that this recovery is rarely a complete recovery. I have learned over the course of my own improvement not to insist on a complete recovery. If I could get to 70 to 80 percent normal I would be ever so thankful! That percentage of recovery would probably mean that some symptoms would remain. I can live with that and I can live well.

A Successful Recovery Process Means the Absence of Expectations

Thinking of chronic conditions only as a curse and a burden narrows your outlook. As a result, you may refuse to look within yourself to find what has been neglected and ignored.

When you begin to see improvement—or even before you see improvement—there is a natural tendency to set expectations about the amounts of time and effort it should take to see improvement. These expectations add pressure and stress to your improvement efforts—as well as a sense of defeat if they aren't met. Without such pressure and stress, an attitude of tolerance and peace can take hold which will facilitate improvement.

Although I've been on a recovery path for the last several years, I still evaluate how I feel physically every day. There has, however, been a big change in my reaction to feeling poorly: rather than viewing my sick feeling as yet another intolerable frustration, I now view it as part of the natural up-and-down cycle of a body that is strengthening slowly but unevenly. When you lessen the intensity of your emotional reactions to being ill, you can better evaluate how you're actually doing physically and stay on track with your improvement efforts.

I believe in total mind-body integration in treating CFS. The purging of stressful thoughts about the illness—and life itself—a form of emotional recovery that is closely linked to physical recovery. This process of releasing expectations is an important element of improvement—and, ultimately, of healing.

Testing Your Limits

Once you feel some level of restored energy, your lifestyle options increase. You may want to restart those activities that you felt obligated to do before you became ill. However, it's difficult to know how much of your pre-illness activities you can tolerate; your tolerance is limited by your ongoing vulnerability to relapse. I don't believe this vulnerability ever disappears, so if you do attempt to resume your pre-illness life, you put yourself at significant risk for symptom flare-ups, if not complete relapse.

Although these potential boundaries of your wellness may be painful reminders of your fragile condition, they can also coax you into a healthier, more balanced life. It's important to tell yourself what the benefits of a more balanced lifestyle are: improved relationships with others, less pressure, more relaxation, longer periods of feeling well, and the release of impossible goals. Remind yourself of these benefits daily, especially in the early phases of improvement.

What Would You Like to Do When You Have Recovered?

This is a critical question that has both an easy immediate answer and a more thoughtful, more measured response. The easy answer: simply resume your old lifestyle. By this point in your reading, you're well aware of the risks of such a course of action. But how do you define and construct a new lifestyle—a new one that is illness-resistant?

One way to envision this is to think of the times in your life when you felt at peace. What were you doing then? Fill in all the details. These times may have involved some kind of hobby or leisure time activity—or perhaps a talent that has withered from disuse. Alternatively, you might have felt at peace during special moments with significant others and close friends or during an uplifting religious or spiritual experience. These are the areas of your life that have suffered most from neglect. Continue to fill in the details of your pleasant memory—and then consider how you might fit it, or something like it, into your life now. You want these peace-producing activities to become a significant part of your life.

The Importance of Healing

Healing is different from cure or recovery. Healing involves restoring a sense of psychic wholeness. You could be cured without necessarily being healed. Healing is a different concept altogether—it involves the creation of a flexible, balanced attitude toward life where the needs of the self are balanced with the needs of others. In the process of healing, you develop and value yourself, not only as an engine of work and sacrifice, but also as a human being with important personal needs. Curing symptoms without healing means that you are much more vulnerable to relapses. A cure without healing will probably be short-lived; your desperation to recapture your pre-illness lifestyle will just deplete your precious energies all over again.

Healing begins when you listen to your body and respect the signals that come from it. For too long your history has been to ignore your body's signals and push onward regardless of the consequences. Respecting signals of exhaustion, pain, and stress allows you to recognize your responsibility to yourself to preserve your health. Healing means that you permit yourself time to preserve your health—and recover as much as possible. You cannot directly control the process of recovery, but you can guide yourself through a healing process that ultimately leads to improvement and perhaps near-recovery. There's a bridge between illness and recovery; it's called "healing."

Resources

To order Dr. Friedberg's professionally prepared relaxation CD or audiocassette tape, please send $19 to:

Fred Friedberg
P.O. Box 456
Kent, CT 06757

(Please specify CD or cassette tape.)

Fibromyalgia

Fibromyalgia Network
    P.O. Box 31750
    Tucson, AZ 85751-1750
    (800) 853-2929
    www.fmnetnews.com

The National Fibromyalgia Association
    www.FMAware.org

Chronic Fatigue Syndrome

CFIDS Association of America, Inc.
P.O. Box 220398
Charlotte, NC 28222-0398
(704) 365-2343
www.cfids.org

The National CFIDS Foundation, Inc.
103 Aletha Road
Needham, MA 02492
(781) 449-3535
Fax: (781) 449-8606
www.ncf-net.org

International Association for Chronic Fatigue Syndrome
www.aacfs.org
An organization of medical research scientists and health professionals dedicated to the study and treatment of CFS.

Co-Cure
www.co-cure.org
A CFS and FM informational Web site and mailing list designed to promote effective distribution and exchange of information between medical/clinical, political, and patient communities.

References

Anonymous. 1999. Quoted from an unidentified Web site.

Assefi, N. P., K. J. Sherman, C. Jacobsen, J. Goldberg, W. R. Smith, and D. Buchwald. 2005. A randomized clinical trial of acupuncture compared with sham acupuncture in fibromyalgia. *Annals of Internal Medicine* 143:16-19.

Barsky, A. J., and J. F. Borus. 1999. Functional somatic syndromes. *Annals of Internal Medicine* 130:910-21.

Behan, P. O., W. M. Behan, and D. Horrobin. 1990. Effect of high doses of essential fatty acids on the postviral fatigue syndrome. *Acta Neurologica Scandinavica* 82:209-16.

Bohr, T. 2000. Fibromyalgia. MSNBC program.

Brown, W. A., A. D. Sirota, R. Niaura, and T. O. Engebretson. 1993. Endocrine correlates of sadness and elation. *Psychosomatic Medicine* 55:458-467.

Buckelew, S. P., B. Huyser, J. E. Hewett, J. C. Parker, J. C. Johnson, R. Conway, and D. R. Kay. 1996. Self-efficacy predicting outcome among fibromyalgia subjects. *Arthritis Care & Research* 9:97-104.

Buckelew, S. P., S. E. Murray, J. E. Hewett, J. Johnson, and B. Huyser. 1995. Self-efficacy, pain, and physical activity among fibromyalgia subjects. *Arthritis Care & Research* 8:43-50.

Campbell, B. 2002. Self Help and CFIDS. *CFIDS Chronicle*, Spring, 20-23.

Cleary, A. 2002. Cortisol as an outcome predictor in cognitive-behavioral treatment of chronic fatigue syndrome. Paper presented at the Conference on Fatigue, Cold Spring Harbor, NY.

Cohen, S. 2005. The Pittsburgh common cold studies: Psychosocial predictors of susceptibility to respiratory infectious illness. *International Journal of Behavioral Medicine* 12:123-131.

Currie, S. R., K. G. Wilson, and D. Curran. 2002. Clinical significance and predictors of treatment response to cognitive-behavior therapy for insomnia secondary to chronic pain. *Journal of Behavioral Medicine* 25:135-153.

Dailey, P. A., G. D. Bishop, I. J. Russell, and E. Fletcher. 1990. Psychological stress and the fibrositis/fibromyalgia syndrome. *Journal of Rheumatology* 17:1380-1385.

Deale, A., T. Chalder, I. Marks, and S. Wessely. 1997. Cognitive behaviour therapy for chronic fatigue syndrome: A randomized controlled trial. *American Journal of Psychiatry* 154:408-414.

De Meirleir, K., C. Bisbal, I. Campine, P. De Becker, T. Salehzada, E. Demettre, and B. Lebleu. 2000. A 37 kDa 2–5A binding protein as a potential biochemical marker for chronic fatigue syndrome. *American Journal of Medicine* 108:99-105.

Elliott, H. 1999. Use of formal and informal care among people with prolonged fatigue: A review of the literature. *British Journal of General Practice* 49:131-134.

Engel, G. L. 1977. The need for a new medical model: A challenge for biomedicine. *Science* 196:129-136.

Field, T. M., W. Sunshe, M. Hernandez-Reif, O. Quintino, S. Schanberg, C. Kuhn, and I. Burman. 1997. Massage therapy effects on depression and somatic symptoms in chronic fatigue syndrome. *Journal of Chronic Fatigue Syndrome* 3:43-52.

Friedberg, F. 1995. *Coping with Chronic Fatigue Syndrome: Nine Things You Can Do*. Oakland, CA New Harbinger.

Friedberg, F. 2002. Does graded activity increase activity?

Friedberg, F., L. Dechene, M. J. McKenzie 2nd, and R. Fontanetta. 2000. Symptom patterns in long-duration chronic fatigue syndrome. *Journal of Psychosomatic Research* 48:59-68.

Fukuda, K., S. E. Straus, I. Hickie, M. C. Sharpe, J. G. Dobbins, and A. Komaroff. 1994. The chronic fatigue syndrome: A comprehensive approach to its definition and study. *Annals of Internal Medicine* 121:953-959.

Garssen, B. 2004. Psychological factors and cancer development: Evidence after 30 years of research. *Clinical Psychology Review* 24:315-338.

Goldenberg, D. L., M. Mayskiy, C. Mossey, R. Ruthazer, and C. Schmid. 1996. A randomized, double-blind crossover trial of fluoxetine and amitriptyline in the treatment of fibromyalgia. *Arthritis and Rheumatism* 39:1852-1859.

Greenberg, M. A., V. L. Dowling, M. S. Hatcher, B. J. Cox, R. E. Marcus, and S. A. Paget. 1999. Emotion-management predicts health outcomes in fibromyalgia. Poster session presented at the annual meeting of the Society of Behavioral Medicine, San Diego, CA.

Heim, C., U. Ehlert, and D. H. Hellhammer. 2000. The potential role of hypocortisolism in the pathophysiology of stress-related bodily disorders. *Psychoneuroendocrinology* 25:1-35.

Hickie, I., and T. Davenport. 1999. The case of Julio: A behavioral approach based on reconstructing the sleep-wake cycle. *Cognitive and Behavioral Practice* 6:442-450.

Holm, J. E., C. Lokken, and T. Cook Myers. 1997. Migraine and stress: A daily examination of temporal relationships in women migraineurs. *Headache* 37:553-558.

Jacobsen, S. 1991. Oral S-adenosylmethione in primary fibromyalgia. Double-blind clinical evaluation. *Scandinavian Journal Of rheumatology* 20:294-302.

Jason, L. A., J. A. Richman, A. W. Rademaker, K. M. Jordan, A. V. Plioplys, R. R. Taylor, W. McCreedy, C. Huang, and S. Plioplys. 1999. A community-based study of chronic fatigue syndrome. *Archives of Internal Medicine* 159:2129-2137.

Jason, L. A., S. R. Torres-Harding, A. W. Carrico, and R. R. Taylor. 2002. Symptom occurrence in persons with chronic fatigue syndrome. *Biological Psychology* 59:15-27.

Kansky, G., and C. Tai. 1999. Ampligen report exposed: Patients duped. *National Forum* 3:8–11.

Kaplan, K. H., D. L. Goldenberg, and M. Galvin-Nadeau. 1993. The impact of a meditation-based stress reduction program on fibromyalgia. *General Hospital Psychiatry* 15:284-289.

Kerns, R. D., R. Rosenberg, and M. C. Jacob. 1994. Anger expression and chronic pain. *Journal of Behavioral Medicine* 17:57-67.

Ketterer, M. W., G. Mahr, and A. D. Goldberg. 2000. Psychological factors affecting a medical condition: Ischemic coronary heart disease. *Journal of Psychosomatic Research* 48:357-367.

Lewis, S., C. L. Cooper, and D. Bennett. 1994. Psychosocial factors and chronic fatigue syndrome. *Psychological Medicine* 24:661-671.

Long, D. M., M. BenDebba, W. S. Torgerson, R. J. Boyd, E. G. Dawson, R. W. Hardy, J. T. Robertson, G. W. Sypert, and C. Watts. 1996. Persistent back pain and sciatica in the United States: Patient characteristics. *Journal of Spinal Disorders* 9:40-58.

Lutgendorf, S. K., M. H. Antoni, G. Ironson, M. A. Fletcher, F. Penedo, A. Baum, N. Schneiderman, and N. Klimas. 1995. Physical symptoms of chronic fatigue syndrome are exacerbated by the stress of Hurricane Andrew. *Psychosomatic Medicine* 57:310-323.

Mannerkorpi, K., B. Nyberg, M. Ahlmen, and C. Ekdahl. 2000. Pool exercise combined with an education program for patients with fibromyalgia syndrome: A prospective, randomized study. *Journal of Rheumatology* 27:2473-2481.

Moldofsky, H. 1993. Sleep and the chronic fatigue syndrome. In *Chronic Fatigue Syndrome*, edited by M. Dawson and T. D. Sabin. Boston: Little, Brown.

Moldofsky, H., P. Scarisbrick, R. England, and H. Smythe. 1975. Musculoskeletal symptoms and non-REM sleep disturbance in patients with "fibrositis syndrome" and healthy subjects. *Psychosomatic Medicine* 34:341.

Nicassio, P. M., K. Schoenfeld-Smith, V. Radojevic, and C. Schuman. 1995. Pain coping mechanisms in fibromyalgia: Relationship to pain and functional outcomes. *Journal of Rheumatology* 22:1552-1558.

Okifuji, A., D. C. Turk, and S. L. Currani. 1999. Anger in chronic pain. Investment of anger targets and intensity. *Journal of Psychosomatic Research* 47:1-12.

Payer, L. 1988. *Medicine and Culture: Varieties of Treatment in the United States, England, West Germany and France.* New York: Holt.

Plioplys, A. V., and S. Plioplys. 1997. Amantadine and L-carnitine treatment of chronic fatigue syndrome. *Neuropsychobiology* 35:16-23.

Prins, J., G. Bleijenberg, E. Bazelmans, L. D. Elving, T. M. deBoo, J. L. Severens, G. J. van der Wilt, P. Spinhoven, and J. W. van der Meer. 2001. Cognitive behavior therapy for chronic fatigue syndrome: A multicentre randomized controlled trial. *Lancet* 357:841-847.

Psychosomatic Medicine. 2001. Practicing meditation can decrease body response to stress. American Psychosomatic Society. McLean, VA.

Ray, C., S. Jefferies, and W. R. C. Weir. 1995. Life-events and the course of chronic fatigue syndrome. *British Journal of Medical Psychology* 68:323-331.

Ray, C., S. Jefferies, and W. R. C. Weir. 1997. Coping and other predictiors of outcome in chronic fatigue syndrome. A 1-year follow up. *Journal of Psychosomatic Research* 43:405-412.

Rossy, L. A., S. P. Buckelew, N. Dorr, K. J. Hagglund, J. F. Thayer, M. J. McIntosh, J. E. Hewett, and J. C. Johnson. 1999. A meta-analysis of fibromyalgia treatment interventions. *Annals of Behavioral Medicine* 21:180-191.

Russell, I. J., J. E. Michalek, J. D. Flechas, and G. E. Abrams. 1995. Treatment of fibromyalgia syndrome with Super Malic: A randomized, double-blind, placebo controlled, crossover pilot study. *Journal of Rheumatology* 22:953-958.

Saltzstein, B. J., G. Wyshak, J. T. Hubbuch, and J. C. Perry. 1998. A naturalistic study of the chronic fatigue syndrome among women in primary care. *General Hospital Psychiatry* 20:307-316.

Sharpe, M., K. Hawton, S. Simkin, C. Surawy, A. Hackmann, I. Klimes, T. Peto, D. Warrell, and V. Seagroatt. 1996. Cognitive behaviour therapy for the chronic fatigue syndrome: A randomized controlled trial. *British Medical Journal* 312:22-26.

Sherman, J. J., D. C. Turk, and A. Okifuji. 2000. Prevalence and impact of posttraumatic stress disorder—like symptoms on patients with fibromyalgia syndrome. *Clinical Journal of Pain* 16:127-134.

Shorter, E. 1995. Sucker-punched again! Physicians meet the disease-of-the-month syndrome. *Journal of Psychosomatic Research* 39:115-118.

Smith, J. C. 1990. *Cognitive-Behavioral Relaxation Training*. New York: Springer.

Sim, J., and N. Adams. 2002. Systematic review of randomized controlled trials of nonpharmacological interventions for fibromyalgia. *Clinical Journal of Pain* 18:324-336.

Spierings E L., A. H. Ranke, and P. C. Honkoop. 2001. Precipitating and aggravating factors of migraine versus tension-type headache. *Headache*. 41:554-8.

Strayer, D. R., W. A. Carter, I. Brodsky, P. C. Cheney, D. Peterson, P. Salvato, C. Thompson, et al. 1994. A controlled clinical trial with a specifically configured RNA drug, poly(I)poly (C12U), in chronic fatigue syndrome. *Clinical Infectious Diseases* 18(Suppl 1):S88-S95.

Suhadolnik, R. J., D. L. Peterson, P. R. Cheney, S. E. Horvath, N. L. Reichenbach, K. O'Brien, V. Lombardi, et al. 1999. Biochemical dysregulation of the 2-5A synthetase/RNase L antiviral defense pathway in chronic fatigue syndrome. *Journal of Chronic Fatigue Syndrome* 5:223-242.

Theorell, T., V. Blomkvist, G. Lindh, and B. Evengard. 1999. Critical life events, infections, and symptoms during the year preceding chronic fatigue syndrome (CFS): An examination of CFS patients and subjects with a nonspecific life crisis. *Psychosomatic Medicine* 61:304-310.

Van Houdenhove, B., E. Neerinckx, P. Onghena, R. Lysens, and H. Vertommen. 2001. Premorbid "overactive" lifestyle in chronic fatigue syndrome and fibromyalgia: An etiological factor or proof of good citizenship? *Journal of Psychosomatic Research* 51:571-576.

Van Houdenhove, B., P. Onghena, E. Neerinckx, and J. Hellin. 1995. Does high "action proneness" make people more vulnerable to chronic fatigue syndrome? A controlled psychometric study. *Journal of Psychosomatic Research* 39:633-640.

Vercoulen, J. H., C. M. Swanink, J. F. Fennis, J. M. Galama, J. W. van der Meer, and G. Bleijenberg. 1996. Prognosis in chronic fatigue syndrome: A prospective study on the natural course. *Journal of Neurology, Neurosurgery & Psychiatry* 60:489-494.

Vercoulen, J. H. M. M., C. M. A. Swanink, F. G. Zitman, G. S. Vreden, and M. P. E. Hoofs. 1996. Randomized, double-blind, placebo-controlled study of fluoxetine in chronic fatigue syndrome. *Lancet* 347:858-862.

Volkmann H., J. Norregaard, S. Jacobsen, B. Danneskiold-Samsoe, G. Knoke, and D. Nehrdich. 1997. Double-blind, placebo-controlled cross-over study of intravenous S-adenosyl-L-methionine in patients with fibromyalgia. *Scandinavian Journal of Rheumatology* 26(3):206-11

Wacogne, C., J. P. Lacoste, E. Guillibert, E. C. Hughes, and C. LeJeunne. 2003. Stress, anxiety, depression and migraine. *Cephalalgia* 23:451-455.

Ware, N. C. 1993. Society, mind, and body in chronic fatigue syndrome: An anthropological view. In *Chronic Fatigue Syndrome*, edited by G. R. Boch and J. Whelan. New York: Wiley.

Warren, G., M. McKendrick, and M. Peet. 1999. The role of essential fatty acids in chronic fatigue syndrome: A case-controlled study of red-cell membrane essential fatty acids (EFA) and a placebo-controlled treatment study. *Acta Neurologica Scandinavica* 99:112-116.

Wearden, A. J., R. K. Morriss, R. Mullis, P. L. Strickland, D. J. Pearson, L. Appleby, I. T. Campbell, and J. A. Morris. 1998. Randomised, double-blind, placebo-controlled treatment trial of fluoxetine and graded exercise for chronic fatigue syndrome. *British Journal of Psychiatry* 172:485-490.

White, K. P., W. R. Nielson, M. Harth, T. Ostbye, and M. Speechley. 2002. Does the label "fibromyalgia" alter health status, function, and health service utilization? A prospective, within-group comparison in a community cohort of adults with chronic widespread pain. *Arthritis and Rheumatism* 47:260-265.

Wolfe, F., H. A. Smythe, M. B. Yunus, R. M. Bennett, C. Bombardier, D. L. Goldenburg, P. Tugwell, et al. 1990. The American College of Rheumatology 1990 criteria for the classification of fibromyalgia. *Arthritis and Rheumatology* 33:160-172.

Wood, G. C., R. P. Bentall, M. Gopfert, M. E. Dewey, and R. H. T. Edwards. 1994. The differential response of chronic fatigue, neurotic and muscular dystrophy patients to experimental psychological stress. *Psychological Medicine* 24:357-364.

Woodward, R. V., D. H. Broom, and D. G. Legge. 1995. Diagnosis in chronic illness: Disabling or enabling—the case of chronic fatigue syndrome. *Journal of the Royal Society of Medicine* 88:325-329.

Fred Friedberg, Ph.D., is a clinical psychologist in practice for 20 years and an assistant professor in the School of Medicine at Stony Brook University, Stony Brook, on Long Island, NY. He has authored two popular books, *Coping with Chronic Fatigue Syndrome* and *Do-It-Yourself Eye Movement Technique for Emotional Healing*. Currently, he is the principal investigator of a five-year behavioral study of chronic fatigue syndrome funded by the National Institutes of Health. His published scientific articles have appeared in *American Psychologist, Journal of Clinical Psychology, Professional Psychology: Research and Practice, Clinical Infectious Diseases, Journal of Neuropsychiatry, Archives of Neurology, Journal of Psychosomatic Research, Cognitive and Behavioral Practice, Journal of Behavior Therapy and Experimental Psychiatry,* and *Journal of Chronic Fatigue Syndrome*. In addition, he has conducted professional workshops for the American Psychological Association, the Association for the Advancement of Behavior Therapy, and the Society of Behavioral Medicine.

Some Other
New Harbinger Titles

Depressed and Anxious, Item 3635 $19.95

Angry All the Time, Item 3929 $13.95

Handbook of Clinical Psychopharmacology for Therapists, 4th edition, Item 3996 $55.95

Writing For Emotional Balance, Item 3821 $14.95

Surviving Your Borderline Parent, Item 3287 $14.95

When Anger Hurts, 2nd edition, Item 3449 $16.95

Calming Your Anxious Mind, Item 3384 $12.95

Ending the Depression Cycle, Item 3333 $17.95

Your Surviving Spirit, Item 3570 $18.95

Coping with Anxiety, Item 3201 $10.95

The Agoraphobia Workbook, Item 3236 $19.95

Loving the Self-Absorbed, Item 3546 $14.95

Transforming Anger, Item 352X $10.95

Don't Let Your Emotions Run Your Life, Item 3090 $17.95

Why Can't I Ever Be Good Enough, Item 3147 $13.95

Your Depression Map, Item 3007 $19.95

Successful Problem Solving, Item 3023 $17.95

Working with the Self-Absorbed, Item 2922 $14.95

The Procrastination Workbook, Item 2957 $17.95

Coping with Uncertainty, Item 2965 $11.95

The BDD Workbook, Item 2930 $18.95

You, Your Relationship, and Your ADD, Item 299X $17.95

The Stop Walking on Eggshells Workbook, Item 2760 $18.95

Conquer Your Critical Inner Voice, Item 2876 $15.95

The PTSD Workbook, Item 2825 $17.95

Hypnotize Yourself Out of Pain Now!, Item 2809 $14.95

Call **toll free, 1-800-748-6273,** or log on to our online bookstore at **www.newharbinger.com** to order. Have your Visa or Mastercard number ready. Or send a check for the titles you want to New Harbinger Publications, Inc., 5674 Shattuck Ave., Oakland, CA 94609. Include $4.50 for the first book and 75¢ for each additional book, to cover shipping and handling. (California residents please include appropriate sales tax.) Allow two to five weeks for delivery.

Prices subject to change without notice.